MW00464232

Podiatry Medical Student Handbook

By Eric Shi, DPM

The most common question of every podiatric medical student is this: "*What book are you using to studying from*?" When I was a student at the College of Podiatric Medicine at Western University of Health Sciences, my mentor and dean of the college, Dr. Lawrence Harkless shared with me that when he was a student, he made 3 x 5 cards of every pathology he saw in clinic and he would carry these cards with him in his pocket wherever he went so he could be constantly reviewing. He recommended I do the same, by breaking down every pathology into the following sections: etiology (ET), epidemiology (EP), risk factors (RF), natural history (NH), diagnosis (DX), and treatment (TX). This manual is my attempt at these 3 x 5 cards. I compiled this material for my self-enrichment for rapid review of material during externships and in preparation for boards and residency interviews. I put it on my iPad and carried it wherever I went during my 3rd and 4th years of podiatry school—the OR, clinic, airport, plane, you name it. I did my best to include as much evidence-based sources as possible—including some of the most landmark foot and ankle articles from Journal of Foot and Ankle Surgery (JFAS), Journal of Bone and Joint Surgery (JBJS), and Foot and Ankle International (FAI). It is by no means an end-all-be-all source for your podiatric knowledge, but a quick review of some of the most high-yield material for externships, boards, and residency interviews.

I hope you find this book helpful. If you find any errors or have any questions, feel free to contact me at pmshandbook@gmail.com.

Happy studying!

Eric Shi, DPM

Podiatric Medical Student Handbook

Diabetes, Infections & Wound Care

Diabetic Foot Ulcer (DFU)

> *"Pressure is the critical quantity that determines the harm done by the force"*
> *-Paul W. Brand, MD*

ET:
1. Repetitive microtrauma (2/2 neuropathy + deformity), cumulative stress
   o Determined by amount of physical activity
2. Continuous pressure (decubitus ulcer)
3. Undetected act of injury (trauma, nail in shoe)
   - Tenderizing the foot (Brand, FAI 2003[1]) depends on:
     o *Pre-ulcerative lesion: once the foot is TENDER (warm, inflamed) a SMALLER stimulus produces LARGER pain.*
       Repetitive, moderate mechanical stress
     o Degree of <u>sensory loss</u>
     o <u>MAGNITUDE</u> of forces
     o <u>QUANTITY</u> of steps to reach inflammation
   - **VIP**: vascular, infection, pressure
   - Chronic wounds:
     o Stuck in inflammatory phase, low mitogenic activity, high protease

EP:
   - Foot ulcers are the #1 reason for hospital admission in diabetics (Lavery et al, Diabetes Care 2006[2])
   - 4-10% in diabetics, 25% lifetime risk (Singh et al, JAMA 2005[3])
   - 1 in 5 of infected ulcers result in amputation (Lavery et al, Clinics in Infectious Disease 2007[4])
   - For every 30 increase in blood sugar = 1 HbA1C = 28% PVD
   - HbA1C > 6.4-7 is diabetic

NH:
1. Amputation leading to increased energy cost of walking, increased O2 consumption (Waters et al, JBJS 1976[5])
2. Mortality due to cardiovascular dz
3. 14 year reduction in life expectancy

5 year mortality rates s/p DFU[6]

	Mortality
DFU w/o BKA	40%
DFU w/ BKA	63%[7]

Risk factors for death: increased age, male gender, peripheral vascular disease and renal disease.

Mortality rates s/p BKA[8]

Years after BKA	Mortality
1 year	18%

---

[1] Brand, Paul W. "Tenderizing the foot." Foot & ankle international 24.6 (2003): 457-461.
[2] Lavery, Lawrence A., et al. "Risk factors for foot infections in individuals with diabetes." Diabetes care 29.6 (2006): 1288-1293.
[3] Singh, Nalini, David G. Armstrong, and Benjamin A. Lipsky. "Preventing foot ulcers in patients with diabetes." Jama 293.2 (2005): 217-228.
[4] Lavery, Lawrence A., et al. "Validation of the Infectious Diseases Society of America's diabetic foot infection classification system." Clinical infectious diseases 44.4 (2007): 562-565
[5] Waters, R. L., et al. "Energy cost of walking of amputees: the influence of level of amputation." The Journal of Bone & Joint Surgery 58.1 (1976): 42-46.
[6] Jupiter, Daniel C., et al. "The impact of foot ulceration and amputation on mortality in diabetic patients. I: From ulceration to death, a systematic review." International wound journal (2015).
[7] Apelqvist J, Larsson J, Agardh CD. Long-term prognosis for diabetic patients with foot ulcers. J Intern Med 1993;233:485 – 91.
[8] Lee JS, Lu M, Lee VS, Russel D, Bahr C, Lee ET. Lower extremity amputation: incidence, risk factors, and mortality in the Oklahoma Indian diabetes study. Diabetes 42:876–882, 1993.

5 years	50%

Energy expenditure increase in patients with BKA vs AKA

Type of amputation	Energy increase
BKA	10-40%
AKA	50-70%

Probability of future amputations s/p BKA

Type of BKA	Chance of BKA in 5 years
Regular BKA	50%
Diabetic BKA	66%

International working group diabetic foot (IWGDF)[9]

IWGDF	Criteria	Likelihood of re-ulceration	Follow up
0	No neuropathy	--	Once a year
1	Neuropathy	2x	Once every 6 months
2a	Neuropathy + PVD	12x	3 months
2b	Neuropathy + deformity (and/or PVD) (pes cavus, contractures 2/2 to neuropathy, collagen glycosylation @ Achilles T)	12x	3 months
3a	History of ulcer	36x	1-3 months
3b	History of amputation	36x	1-3 months

Wagner/University of Texas classification[10]

	Wagner A-neuropathic B-ischemic C-neuroischemic	UT	UT
0	Pre-ulcerative	Pre-ulcerative	A = noninfected / nonischemic
1	Superficial (partial or full thickness)	*Superficial* (partial or full thickness)	B = infected
2	Deep to tendon, capsule, bone, ligament	Deep to tendon or capsule	C = ischemic
3	2 + abscess or active infection	Deep to bone or joint, (osteomyelitis, abscess, septic joint)	D = infection + ischemia

---

[9] Lavery et al, Effectiveness of the Diabetic Foot Risk Classification System of the International Working Group on the Diabetic foot, Diabetes Care 2001, 24; 8:1442-47

[10] Lavery, Lawrence A., David G. Armstrong, and Lawrence B. Harkless. "Classification of diabetic foot wounds." The Journal of foot and ankle surgery 35.6 (1996): 528-531.

| 4 | Forefoot gangrene | | |
| 5 | Rearfoot gangrene | | |

Pathophysiology (Brownlee, Diabetes 2005[11])
1. Polyol pathway (sorbitol-aldose reuctase pathway)
   a. bad pathway!
   b. **Aldose reductase** in the presence of X5 glucose reduces it into sorbitol, which then becomes fructose. Accumulation of sorbitol and fructose, which can't cross cell membrane, increase osmotic pressure.
   c. Decreased NADH, decreased reduced glutathione, increased oxidative stress
2. Production of Advanced Glycation End product (AGE)
   a. AGE binds to RAGE found on cells of the body —> inflammatory cytokines, decreased mobility, rigidity
      i. inflammation —> decreased collagen synthesis, inhibition of keratinocyte differentiation
   b. AGE modifies albumin
3. PKC activation
4. Increased hexosamine pathway
5. Immunocompromised-decreased neutrophil activity, decreased cytokines, decreased immunoglobulin and complement function, decreased antigen presentation by monocytes
   a. Hypoglycemia (<80) and hyperglycemia (>150) increases surgical infection
   b. 3x surgical risk for infection
   c. Don't do surgery on a patient with a HbA1C > 8
6. Non-enzymatic glycosylation
   a. Tendons-decreased elasticity and tensile strength
      i. Equinovarus deformity
   b. Joints-subluxation, stiffness, instability
   c. Skin-glycosylation of keratin
   d. Bone
7. Chronic inflammation
   a. weakened leukocyte adhesion, chemotaxis of cytokines
8. Vasculopathy
   a. Micro-vascular disease-retinopathy, neuropathy, nephropathy
      i. Thickened basement membrane—>poor diffusion
   b. Macro-vascular disease-PVD, CAD, stroke, claudication, rest pain
      i. oxidation of LDL
   c. Functional micro-vascular-ANS, gastroparesis, impotence
   d. Metabolic syndrome-HTN, hyperlipidemia, smoking, obesity, impaired glucose tolerance (IGT), insulin resistance (IR)
9. Nephropathy —> CKD —> decreased EPO production —> anemia
10. Bone healing
    a. 1 in 4 diabetics will have bone healing complication
       i. HbA1C > 7 increases bone healing complication 3X
       ii. Neuropathy is the #1 factor for bone healing complication
          1. Lack of neuropeptide release up-regulates **osteoclasts** and down-regulates **osteoblasts**

Effects of hyperglycemia:

Increased	Decreased
Sorbitol & Fructose <—CULPRIT	NO
ROS	Reduced glutathione
NADH/FADH	eNOS
AGE	NADH
Pro-inflammatory cytokines	

---

[11] Brownlee, Michael. "The pathobiology of diabetic complications a unifying mechanism." Diabetes 54.6 (2005): 1615-1625.

Superoxide production	

CP:
Types of Ulcers

	Appearance	Other
Neuropathic	Granular base = beefy red Fibrotic base = yellow Necrotic base = black	-Factors affecting healing: "**VIP**"—vascular/infection/pressure -Located on WB surface -Hyperkeratotic border
Ischemic/arterial insufficiency ulcer	Pale, **NON-granular base**, necrosis, "punched out", minimal drainage	DISTAL to medial malleolus -Absent pulses -Irregular edge
Neuroischemic	Medial 1st MTPJ, lateral 5th MTPJ	-most difficult/challenging to treat
Venous stasis ulcer/stasis dermatitis	Scaly, shallow, granulating base, venous weeping, oozing, hemosiderin deposits	PROXIMAL to medial malleolus, pulses palpable, rounded edge, stasis dermatitis

Other ulcerations

Ulcer appearance	Etiology, TX
Circular, sub 1st	ET: sagittal plane forces TX: TAL, flexor tenotomy, Jones tenosuspension
Oval, sub 5th	ET: transverse/frontal plane (SHEAR forces) TX: TAT lenthening
Hallux IPJ ulcer, "pinch callus"	ET: hallux limitus/rigidus, hypermobile 1st ray leading to pronation TX: Keller

- Rim of hyperkeratotic tissue surrounding ulcer ("edge effect": greater rim of hyperkeratosis = improper offloading)
- Skin sloughing
- Fat necrosis
- Emphysema: soft tissue air-like density
- DPRESTO + BBMP: **D**rainage, **P**robe to bone, **R**edness, **E**dema, **S**inus tracking, **T**emperature, **O**dor + **B**ase, **B**order, **M**easurement, **P**eriwound skin
  - o Cellulitis-erythema that does not resolve with elevation
  - o Sinus: soft tissue tract feeding from ulcer
  - o Fluctuance: fluid/abscess
  - o Induration: hard mass indicating inflammation
  - o Full thickness or partial thickness
  - o Drainage-purulence/serous, depth (more deep = long standing)

Drainage	Serous, sanguinous, purulent,
Base	Granular base = beefy red, Fibrotic base = yellow, Necrotic base = black
Border	Hyperkeratotic, macerated, necrotic, clean, bleeding, epithelial, undermining, tunneling
Periwound skin	Normal, erythema, streaking, stasis change, trophic change

Depth	Skin, superficial fascia, deep fascia (muscle), periosteum, bone

PEDIS system (by IWGDF)[12]

Acronym	Description
Perfusion	Arterial supply
Extent	Area
Depth	Tissue loss
Infection	
Sensation	Neuropathy

DX:
- Constitutional symptoms
- Laboratory tests
- CBC, WBC, ESR, CRP, procalcitonin
- Results may be blunted due to immunosuppression 2/2 to diabetes

Cultures:
o Soft tissue culture and sensitivity
    o ONLY if there are signs of infection—culture as deep as possible
        ▪ Soft tissue culture >> swab
        ▪ Cleanse, debride wound, obtain tissue from deep tissue
        ▪ soft tissue biopsy > swab
    o Gram stain, aerobic/anaerobes, fungal
        ▪ Majority are polymicrobial
    o **"Critical colonization"/"increased bioburden"**: >100,000 colony forming units (CFU) per gram of tissue in the absence of clinical infection
    o >30 days increase infection
    o earlier detection than XR
    o PCR ($$$) > plate culture
o Blood culture

Microbiology: diabetic foot ulcer culture results

Culture	Gram stain	Clinical appearance
Staph	gram + cocci in cluster, catalase + coagulase +: **S. Aureus** coagulase -: **S. Epi**	**purulence, localized erythema**
Strep	gram + cocci in chains/paired, catalse - group B strep = **Strep agalactiae** group A strep = **Strep pyogenes**	**NO purulence**, GAS = soft tissue emphysema spreads widely along tissue planes, **ascending lymphangitis**
Peptostreptococcus	gram + cocci, anaerobe	soft tissue emphysema, anaerobes are 3% of all DFU
Corynebacterium diptheriae	gram + rod, aerobic	
ALL clostridium: (perfringens, dificile, tetani)	gram + rod with spores, anaerobe	**Clostridium perfringens**: soft tissue emphysema

---

[12] Cavanagh PR et al, Nonsurgical Strategies for Healing and Preventing Recurrence of Diabetic Foot Ulcers, Foot Ankle Clinics, 2006, 735-743

Culture	Gram stain	Clinical appearance
PECKSS Pseudomonas E.coli Klebsiella Shigella Salmonella Vibrio Enterobacter	gram - rod with pilli, aerobic	
Bacteriodes Fragilis	gram - rod, anaerobe	Soft tissue emphysema, distinctive malodor anaerobes are 3% of all DFU
Neisseria gonorrhea	gram - cocci, aerobic	
Treponema pallidum, borrelia burgdorferi	Spirochetes	

Imaging:
- Radiograph
  - XR to rule out soft tissue emphysema
    - ***ANKLE VIEW XR TO R/O GAS***
- CT
  - LEG CT TO R/O GAS

TX:
Pearls:
- #1 priority: best functional outcome/well-being of patient.
  - Usually wound closure, can also include amputation.
- Cannot offload a rigid deformity!
- Biofilm-hydrated matrix of proteins and polysaccharides that encompass a polymicrobial collection of cells
  - IMPORTANCE OF GOOD DEBRIDEMENT OF NECROTIC TISSUE
  - adhere to necrotic bony surface or implants (stainless steel) in a sporelike state. Titanium implants > stainless steel
  - resistant to antibiotics and host defenses
    - body exerts chronic inflammatory response
    - permanent until the affected surface is removed

Prevention:
- Follow-up every 2 months-surveillance (glycemic control, callus debridement (Murray 1996)
  - Monitor foot by checking for lesions, foot temperature
- Check foot TEMPERATURE at bedtime (Brand[13])
- Equip patient with simple skin temperature device (Armstrong[14])
  - Examining foot with mirror offers no benefit compared to general diabetic foot education alone.

TX steps:
Quality of life is influenced more by ability to heal the wound than treatment modality. In other words, to increase quality of life, do whatever it takes (TCC) to heal the wound! (Armstrong et al, JFAS 2008[15])

- Debridement
  - Sharp, mechanical, autolytic
  - Minimize bioburden-prevent infection
- Activity modification
  - decrease the number of steps
- Acute pressure relief (offload): NOT POST-OP SHOE

[13] Brand, Paul W. "Tenderizing the foot." Foot & ankle international 24.6 (2003): 457-461
[14] Armstrong, David G., et al. "Skin temperature monitoring reduces the risk for diabetic foot ulceration in high-risk patients." The American journal of medicine 120.12 (2007): 1042-1046
[15] Armstrong, David G., et al. "Quality of life in healing diabetic wounds: does the end justify the means?." The Journal of Foot and Ankle Surgery 47.4 (2008): 278-282.

- o TCC for 5-8 weeks to offload pressure (Caputo et al, NEJM 1994[16])
- o Only used by 2-6%
- o TCC increases the contact area on plantar foot
  - ▪ PROS: Heals ~85% of all wounds
  - ▪ CONS: High recurrence rate of ulcer
    - Need to surgically correct the deformity
    - Even proper follow up will not prevent recurrences
    - Expensive $$$
    - Risk abrasion, swelling from cast
  - ▪ Instant TCC: (plaster over CAM boot, forced compliance) just as effective as regular TCC
  - ▪ CAM boot: better forefoot offloading pressures than TCC (Gutekunst et al[17])
- o Special padding
  - ▪ "Football dressing" for plantar forefoot wounds
- **Accomodate: protective footwear (DM shoes)**
  - o Custom orthopedic shoes will NOT prevent recurrences
  - o avoid pressure points—evenly re-distributes pressres across plantar foot
  - o Computer-designed insoles determined by insole plantar pressure measuring device
  - o DM shoes=extra depth, wide toe box, plastizote insert, stretch canvas for edema, Velcro strap if unable to tie shoe
- **Surgery**
  - o ONLY for REDUCIBLE deformities
  - o Tendon lengthening-WEAKEN deforming force, NOT increase ROM
- **Re-vascularization (PAD/ischemia)**
  - o consult vascular surgeon if needed

Nonhealing ulcer:
- Anything >6 months
- <50% REDUCTION IN 1 MONTH= UNLIKELY HEALING BY 12 WEEKS, NEED ADJUNCTIVE THERAPY (Sheehan et al, Diabetes Care 2003[18])
- Healing determined by etiology more than size (Zimny et al, 2002[19])

ET:
- Pressure (chronic mechanical trauma) is #1 reason
- Malnutrition (albumin—corrected albumin 2/2 Ca2+)
- Smoking
- Cancer (SCC, Marjolin ulcer)
- Vascular disease
- Infection
- Pyoderma gangrenosum 2/2 pathergy

DX: punch biopsy
TX:
Nutrition
- Zinc, vitamin C, vitamin A, 90g protein/day
Adjunctive therapy
Good evidence: (Cochrane 2010)
1) Hyperbaric oxygen therapy[20] (HBOT), the "kitchen sink"
PROS:
- Good for hypoxic ulcers (DM or arterial insufficiency) with TcPO2 < 50mmHg
- O2 dissolves in the plasma to oxygenate the hypoxic area
- increases perfusion of Abx

---

[16] Caputo, Gregory M., et al. "Assessment and management of foot disease in patients with diabetes." New England Journal of Medicine 331.13 (1994): 854-860
[17] Gutekunst, David J., et al. "Removable cast walker boots yield greater forefoot off-loading than total contact casts." Clinical Biomechanics 26.6 (2011): 649-654.
[18] Sheehan, Peter, et al. "Percent change in wound area of diabetic foot ulcers over a 4-week period is a robust predictor of complete healing in a 12-week prospective trial." Diabetes care 26.6 (2003): 1879-1882.
[19] Zimny, Stefan, Helmut Schatz, and Martin Pfohl. "Determinants and estimation of healing times in diabetic foot ulcers." Journal of Diabetes and its Complications 16.5 (2002): 327-332
[20] Löndahl, Magnus, et al. "Hyperbaric oxygen therapy facilitates healing of chronic foot ulcers in patients with diabetes." Diabetes care 33.5 (2010): 998-1003

- toxic to anaerobes
- increases phagocytosis
- Angiogenesis, antimicrobial, fibroblast production, collagen synthesis, epithelial closure

CONS:
- Expensive, long time (60 hours)
- For refractory ulcers only

2) Negative pressure wound therapy (NPWT) (Wagner 3 or 4)
3) Surgery (to correct structural deformity)
   a. For chronic non healing wounds **with** good vascular status
   b. High risk of infection at surgical site in diabetics
   c. <u>TAL/gastroc recession</u>
      i. Not enough to do on its own
      ii. Rigid rocker decreases plantar pressure (Van Schie et al, FAI 2000[21])
   d. <u>Sesamoidectomy</u>
      i. SE: decreased 1st MTPJ ROM, pain, IPJ contracture
   e. <u>Cavus tendon balancing procedure</u>

<u>Poor evidence:</u>

"It's not what you put on, it's what you take off"

Advanced wound care products: LACK OF STRONG EVIDENCE TO JUSTIFY PROCESS OF WOUND CARE >> PRODUCT OF WOUND CARE
- Products to correct wound biochemistry
  o Platelet-derived topical growth factors (becaplermin)
  o Basic fibroblast growth factor (bFGF)
    - thousands of GF required for wound healing, current products (Regranex) only replace one
    - half life? concentration? mimic real wound healing?
  o Bioengineered skin equivalent/ collagen containing matrix
    - Mesenchymal stem cell (MSC)—amnion and chorion
      - Paracrine function-angiogenic and osteoinductive
      - Non-inflammatory
      - Amnion has 3 week lifespan
  o BM derived stem cells
  o Devitalized allograft
  o Cellular autologous and allogenic skin substitute
- Electromagnetic lasers, shockwaves, ultrasound

Surgery
- I&D vs amputation
  o Packing strips or drain placement
- Vascular consult if vascular compromise
- Delayed primary closure (DPC) for active infection
- Antibiotics
  o Oral or IV
  o Antibiotic impregnated beads
    - high concentration of antibiotics (200x IV Abx)
    - Antibiotic has to be **heat STABLE**, broad spectrum, low allergen (AMINOGLYCOSIDE: gentamycin, tobramycin, vancomycin, clindamycin)
    - PMMA (polymethylmethacrylate)
      - 1:5 (Abx:PMMA) ratio
      - second surgery to remove beads.
    - Calcium sulfate
      - Biodegradable
    - Formation of seroma (inflammatory mediators) in bone cavity

Infection treatment
1) Empiric treatment

Type of infection	Treatment

---

[21] van Schie, Carine, et al. "Design criteria for rigid rocker shoes." Foot & Ankle International 21.10 (2000): 833-844

Non-severe infection, WITHOUT recent antibiotic therapy	Aerobic gram + cocci
Severe infection AND/OR recent antibiotic therapy	Broad spectrum therapy
	Cover MRSA or pseudomonas if risk factors

2) Definitve therapy
- Based on results of C&S and patient's clinical response to empirical regimen

IDSA Treatment Guidelines[22]

Severity	Clinical manifestations of infection	Treatment	PEDIS grade
Uninfected	no signs/symptoms of infection		1
Mild	superficial tissue (skin and subcut): ERYTHEMA <2cm around ulcer	Topical or PO for 1-2 weeks	2
Moderate	deeper tissue (abscess, OM, septic arthritis, fasciits), ERYTHEMA >2cm, lymphatic streaking	IV/PO for 1-3 weeks ADMIT if PAD or lack home support	3
Severe	SIRS criteria	ADMIT IV for 2-4 weeks, can transition to PO	4
Amputation	S/P resection	**clean margins**: IV/PO 2-5 days **residual soft tissue**: IV/PO 2-4 weeks **residual bone**: IV—>PO 4-6 weeks	

Systemic infection

Systemic infection	Criterion
SIRS	(>/= 2 of: temp >38 (>100.4, <96.8), HR >90, RR >20 (PaCO2 <32), WBC >12)
Sepsis	SIRS + source
Severe Sepsis	Sepsis + organ dysfunction/hypotension/hypoperfusion (lactic acidosis, SBP < 90, SBP drop >40 of normal)
Septic Shock	Severe sepsis + hypotension despite fluid resuscitation

MRSA infection
CP:
- no clinical or outcome difference between MRSA and MSSA[23]

TX:
Empirical treatment against MRSA only in 3 conditions:
- history of MRSA
- local prevalence of MRSA colonization or MRSA infection is "high"
- clincially severe infection (sepsis)

Severity of infection	Antimicrobial therapy

[22]Lipsky, Benjamin A., et al. "2012 Infectious Diseases Society of America clinical practice guideline for the diagnosis and treatment of diabetic foot infections." Clinical infectious diseases 54.12 (2012): e132-e173

[23] Zenelaj, Besa, et al. "Do Diabetic Foot Infections With Methicillin-Resistant Staphylococcus aureus Differ From Those With Other Pathogens?." The international journal of lower extremity wounds (2014): 1534734614550311.

Mild	Doxycycline, minocycline, Bactrim, clindamycin, +/- rifampin
Moderate/severe	Linezolid, vancomycin, daptomycin, tigecycline, ceftaroline, televancin

Gas Gangrene, myonecrosis, clostridial myonecrosis, non-clostridial myonecrosis (most common)

A rapidly progressing infection, traditionally clostridium

ET:
- Clostridium perfringens, producing a potent extracellular toxin—> rapid progression
- Group A strep (GAS)-most gas gangrene not clostridium (Brucata et al JFAS 2014)[24]
- Non-clostridium species—> have a slower course
- Post-traumatic, post-operative

RF: DM—greatest risk, PVD

CP:
- SIRS criteria —> sepsis —> septic shock —> kidney failure —> death
- pain out of proportion, severe erythema, necrotic skin. Soft tissue crepitus, painful edema, bullae, serosanguinous drainage, malodor. Altered mental status, shock
- Incubation period usually < 24 hours (usually 7 hours) but can be up to 6 weeks.
- Clinical deterioration can occur within hours

DX:
- IDSA guidelines: cultures confirming Clostridium species

XR: soft tissue emphysema—not always present with gas gangrene, does not confirm diagnosis
- CT-higher sensitivity

TX:
- SURGICAL EMERGENCY, remove necrotic tissue, amputation
- hyperbaric oxygen
- Medical treatment: 10-24 million units of PEN G, clindamycin also useful

Necrotizing Fasciitis, group A beta hemolytic strep (GABS) gangrene, "flesh-eating" bacteria, Fournier's gangrene (peri-anal area)

Infection of superficial, subcutaneous, and deeper tissues-fat and muscle fascia

ET: strep pyogenes, MRSA, staph aureus, group A strep, clostridium perfringens,

RF: immunosuppression, DM, IVDU, PVD

CP:
- RAPID PROGRESSION
- red/purple—>blue/grey patchy skin
- hemorrhagic bullae, gangrene, skin anesthesia
- Pain out of proportion
- +/- soft tissue emphysema, crepitus
- **Systemic symptoms**: fever, tachycardia, neurological deficiencies
- Intra-op:
  - o dish water soap appearance
  - o "finger test"-poke fascia and separates into planes, minimal resistance to finger dissection

DX:
- LRINEC score (Laboratory Risk Indicator for Necrotizing Fasciitis) distinguishes from cellulitis
  - o glucose, CRP, WBC, hemoglobin, sodium, creatinine, glucose

Score	Risk	Risk for necrotizing fasciitis
</= 5	Low	<50%
6-7	Moderate	50-75%
>/=8	High	>75%

TX:
- Surgical emergency—surgical debridement indicated
- 1.2 million U/day PEN G
- Zosyn, Vancomycin, clindamycin

---

[24] Brucato, Maryellen P., Krupa Patel, and Obinna Mgbako. "Diagnosis of Gas Gangrene: Does a Discrepancy Exist between the Published Data and Practice." The Journal of Foot and Ankle Surgery 53.2 (2014): 137-140.

Erysipelas

ET: acute superficial form of cellulitis involving the dermal lymphatics
CP:
- Swollen lymph glands near cellulitis
- Red streaking

IDSA Empiric Antibiotic Regimen[25]:

☒ caution renal failure

	Mild infection	Moderate infection
MSSA	**PO:** Cephalexin 500mg PO QID **IV:** Ancef 2g IV Q4	Unasyn ®
MSSA + anaerobes	**PO:** Augmentin ® 875mg PO BID	Ertapenem
MSSA + ESBL		Imipenem/cilistatin
MRSA	**PO:** Doxycycline, Daptomycin Bactrim, Clindamycin 300mg PO TID (renal failure) **IV:** Clindamycin 900mg IV Q6	Vancomycin, linezolid
Pseudomonas	Zosyn (piperacillin/tazobactam)	
MRSA + pseudomonas	Vancomycin + Zosyn, OR Clindamycin+ Ciprofloxacin (PCN allerg) Vanco requires C&S unless one of risk factors: 1) Hx MRSA 2) Recent (3 months) hospitalization or > weeks 3) Nursing home 4) IVDU	
Recent Abx use (past month)	Cover for gram negative bacilli Fluoroquinolones, aminoglycoside	

Wound Care
Wound dressings Summary

Category	Product	Description
Autolytic debridement	Unna boot, Hydrogel ®, Medihoney ®	Creates moist occlusive environment for **dry/necrotic wounds**, autolytic debridement by body's own phagocytes **Unna Boot**-compression and lotion to promote healing **Medihoney ®**-low pH, moist environment —> mild autolytic debridement by liquefying and softening necrotic tissue
Alginates	Aquacel ®	Made from seaweed, highly absorbent for exudative wounds, bacteriostatic, hemostatic
Films	Tegaderm ®, Telfa	Low adherence
Foams/hydrocolloid	Mepilex ®, Duoderm ®,	Adhesive dressing to create moist environment for fibrinolysis, angiogenesis, and wound healing

---

[25] Lipsky, Benjamin A., et al. "2012 Infectious Diseases Society of America clinical practice guideline for the diagnosis and treatment of diabetic foot infections." Clinical infectious diseases 54.12 (2012): e132-e173.

Low Adherence	Xeroform ®, Adaptic ®, Owens silk,	Keep wounds moist
Enzymatic/chemical debridement	Accuzyme ®, Santyl ®	**Santyl ®**-collagenase—removes fibrotic tissue
Mechanical debridement	Hydrotherapy (Versajet ®), wet to dry dressings	Wet to dry dressings with saline
Silver nitrate		chemically caustic agent used to break down hyper granular wounds so that epithelial borders can touch and close
Scar treatment	Mederma ®	Onion extract

Biologics Summary

Graft name	Material	Other
Apligraf®	• Neonatal foreskin • Bovine collagen	-Epidermal and dermal layer[26] -first FDA approved product for use in DFU -Growth factors and matrix proteins to stimulate proliferation/differentiation -Cons: $$$, shelf life of 10 days -**type 1 collagen and ECM** to stimulate production of cytokines and growth factors
Dermagraft®	• Neonatal foreskin • Polyglactin mesh scaffold	-**collagen and ECM** Dermal layer (fibroblast derived)
TheraSkin ®	Allograft	Epidermis, dermis, ECM
Prisma ®	collagen and cellulose	-**collagen** -becomes a gel in contact with exudate, antibacterial barrier
Acell ®	porcine urinary bladder matrix	-Growth factor[27] -Collagen -epithelial basement membrane (ECM)
Integra ®	Collagen bilayer matrix • Silicone outer layer (functions as epidermis) • Shark chondroitin 6 sulfate & bovine type 1 collagen (functions as dermis)	-**Acellular** scaffold -once dermis forms, follow with STSG -Good for deeper surgically created wounds (patients considering NPWT)
Graftjacket®	Human dermis	**Acellular** scaffold (ECM)
Oasis ®	Porcine small intestine submucosa matrix	**Acellular** scaffold (ECM)

---

[26] Zaulyanov, Larissa, and Robert S. Kirsner. "A review of a bi-layered living cell treatment (Apligraf®) in the treatment of venous leg ulcers and diabetic foot ulcers." Clinical interventions in aging 2.1 (2007): 93
[27] Brown B, Lindberg K, Reing J, Stolz DB, Badylak SF. The basement membrane component of biologic scaffolds derived from extracellular matrix. Tissue Eng 2006;12:519–26.

Primatrix ®	fetal bovine dermis	**Acellular** scaffold (ECM)
Regranex ® (Becaplermin gel)	PDGF (platelet derived growth factors)	Granular, **good blood flow**
Grafix®, Ovation®	Amniotic membrane (cryopreserved)	• Mesoderm/epithelial cells, (ECM)[28] • Growth factors • MSC
Amniox ®	Amniotic membrane and umbilical cord (cryopreserved)	• Mesoderm/epithelial cells, (ECM) • Growth factors • MSC
Epifix ®	Amniotic membrane (dehydrated)	• Mesoderm/epithelial cells, (ECM) • Growth factors • MSC

- Apligraf application
    - Sharp debridement of the wound
    - Cut graft to the right size, mesh with scalpel
    - Secure graft with steri strips, cover with adaptic
    - Document lot #, expiration date, how much was discarded

Use of Biologics Algorithm (Garwood et al, 2015[29])

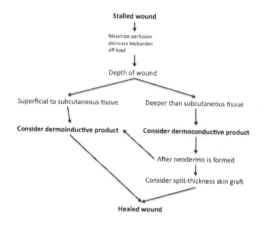

Topical Antimicrobials

---

[28] Lavery, Lawrence A., et al. "The efficacy and safety of Grafix® for the treatment of chronic diabetic foot ulcers: results of a multi-centre, controlled, randomised, blinded, clinical trial." International wound journal 11.5 (2014): 554-560.

[29] Garwood, Caitlin S., John S. Steinberg, and Paul J. Kim. "Bioengineered Alternative Tissues in Diabetic Wound Healing." Clinics in podiatric medicine and surgery 32.1 (2015): 121-133.

Product	Description
Iodosorb/iodoform (cadexomer iodine)	A cicatrizant—promotes healing via formation of scar tissue
Silvadene, silvasorb	Silver sulfadiazine, caution: silver allergy, MACERATION
Betadine	Drys out wound can kill cells at high concentration/long term use
Triple antibiotic ointment (bacitracin)	
Dakins * solution (sodium hypochlorite)	can kill cells at high concentration/long term use

Stages of skin healing or wound healing
Complete healing @ 6-12 months

Phase	Cellular and bio-physiologic events	Time
0) Hemostasis	1) Vascular constriction 2) Platelet aggregation, degranulation, fibrin formation (thrombus)	5-10 minutes
1) Inflammation (substrate/lag phase)	1) Neutrophil/monocyte/lymphocyte migrate to wound site 2) Monocyte differentiation into macrophage *Chronic wounds get stuck in this phase*	1 week
2) Proliferation (fibroplasia, epithelialization, repair phase)	1) Regrowth of epithelial tissue over wound 2) Angiogenesis 3) Collagen synthesis by myofibroblast 4) ECM formation	1-3 week
3) Remodeling (maturation phase)	1) Deposition of matrix materials 2) Collagen remodeling (can last for years)—macrophage debride randomly arranged collagen fibers 3) Vascular maturation and regression	>3 weeks - 1 year

- Types of wound closure
  - o Primary-sutures, linear scar, fastest
    - ▪ Leave sutures in DM patients for twice as long as normal patients (leave nylon sutures x4 wks)
  - o Delayed primary (DPC)-infected wound left open for infection to pass then closed primarily.
    - ▪ Close when wound is granulating and clean
  - o Secondary-left open to granulate bottom up
    - ▪ Wound VAC assist
    - ▪ Primary closure or DPC is ideal
    - ▪ Longer recovery
    - ▪ Allowing large amount of wounds to heal by secondary closure could mean poor decision making
- Healed wound documentation: "wound has fully epithelialized"

Split Thickness skin graft (STSG), autograft
- includes epidermis and various amounts of dermis
- GOLD STANDARD- "next best skin is nearest skin"
- Flaps: bi-lobed, transpositional, V-Y, rotational, rhomboid
- % viable cells: 100 - age

	Thickness	Use
Thin	up to 0.012	temporary coverage of large wounds

Intermediate	0.013-0.016	versatile
Thick	0.017-0.020	WB areas

Skin Graft healing

	Description	Time period
Plasmatic	fibrin layer to anchor graft to recipient	1-2 days
Inosculation	revascularization	2+ days
Reorganization	collagenation, remodeling	weeks-months
Re-innervation		weeks-months

Reasons for failure: #1: seroma, #2: hematoma due to disruption of recipient interface, lack of vasculature, infection, motion at graft site

Osteomyelitis (OM), diabetic foot osteomyelitis (DFO)
- Infection of <u>bone</u> and <u>marrow</u>
  - Infective periostitis-periosteum only
  - Infective osteitis-periosteum + cortex

Waldvogel and Lew Classification for Osteomyelitis
- **Acute**-SYSTEMIC signs of infection, hematogenous
  - from onset of bone infection UNTIL bone becomes necrotic
- **Subacute**-infection not completely eliminated (bone abscess, Garre's)
- **Chronic**-SUBACUTE signs of infection
  - >6 months
    - continuous low grade infection with NECROTIC bone

UTMB Staging system for Osteomyelitis (Cierny-Mader[30])

	Anatomic type
1	Medullary OM
2	Superficial OM
3	Localized OM
4	Diffuse OM
	Host:
A	Good immune system
B	Compromised immune system
C	Not a surgical candidate
	Systemic factors:
	malnutrition, renal failure, DM, age, immunosuprresion, etc

ET:
- Direct extension: penetration into bone

---

[30] A clinical staging system for adult osteomyelitis. CORR. 2003; (414): 7-24

- Pediatric OM: hematogenous spread (children with open physes)
  - **Infant**-open communication between metaphysis and epiphysis
  - **Child**-no communication between metaphysis and epiphysis
  - **Adult**-no physis
- Postoperative

Common microbiology of osteomyelitis, septic arthritis

Bacteria	Susceptible group
Staph aureus	Most common overall
Staph aureus, strep, anaerobes, pseudomonas	IVDU/Diabetics
HiB, GBS	Pediatrics
Coag negative staph	Foreign body
Salmonella	Sickle cell
Aspergillus, MAC, candida albicans	Immunocompromised
N. Gonorrhea	Sexually active, <30 y.o.

RF: Diabetes, PVD, history of infection/amputation, LOPS
CP:
- Subtypes:
  - **Acute**-dx within 2 weeks of onset of symptoms
  - **Subacute**-dx 2 wks after
  - **Chronic**-dx 1 month after, >6 months of infection
- No such thing as "cure" because infection can remain dormant

DX:
- Clinical suspicion: inflammation, purulent discharge, nonhealing wound
- Laboratory test-ESR/CRP
  - Non specific (in the presence of Charcot foot)
  - Very high ESR (70-80) highly suggests OM
- Bone biopsy (gold standard)
  - ideally performed 2 wks Abx free
  - mixed technique: surgical biopsy vs fine needle vs marrow aspirate
  - histology vs microbiolgy
  - Indicated:
    - Desire for early absolute diagnosis to justify treatment
    - Uncertain dx of OM (bias due to pathologist)
    - Inadequate soft tissue cultures
    - Failed empiric ABx therapy
    - Using highly selective ABx

Bone biopsy results

	Bone biopsy findings
OM	necrotic bone
Charcot	shards of bone

- Probe to bone test (PTB):
  - Perform in ALL open wounds
  - Varied positive predictive value
  - Positive predictive value depends on the type of population you are treating:
- Populations with high chance of OM (severe infection) will have higher PPV
- Populations with low chance of OM (outpatient setting) will have lower PPV but high NPV

Validity of Probe to bone test: Grayson[31] vs Lavery[32] vs Shone[33]

Study	Percentage	Population
Grayson (1995)	89% positive predictive value	severe infections
Lavery & Armstrong (2007)	57% positive predictive value 98% negative predictive value	all wounds *"a better test of exclusion in the clinical setting"*
Shone (2006)	53% positive predictive value 85% negative predictive value	all wounds

Imaging
- Preferred: MRI (most sensitive & specific) + bone biopsy
  - T2/STIR: HYPER-intense signal
  - T1: HYPO-intense signal
  - MRI: high sensitivity, but not specific—confusion with charcot/AVN
  - Skewed results 2/2 ischemia
  - False positive: unexplained lucencies noted as marrow edema[34]
- Radiograph
  - **Takes 2 weeks (30-60% bone loss) before x-ray changes visible
    - 2 weeks for osseous washout of minerals
    - can even take >2wks for XR changes
    - Role of nuclear medicine/MRI
- PET/CT-expensive, but may be future of imaging
- Ultrasound-just as useful as XR or MRI, but user-dependant

Bone scan

Type of scan	Details	Positive
Technesium/Tech99/"True" bone scan	-measures osteoblast activity of (hydroxyapatite), NOT infection -intiial injection of radioisotope 1) Flow-angiogram (immediate) 2) Blood pool-hyperemia or ischemia (5-10 minutes), areas of inflammation 3) Delayed phase-rate of bone metabolism (3-4 hours), **positive-OM, negative-cellulitis** 4) Diagnosis-greater bone activity-OM (24 hours)	"Functional" test: any METABOLIC bone activity/remodeling—normal bone growth (ephiphyseal plate), fracture, tumor, charcot, gout
Indium/Indium 111 oxime/WBC scan	ACUTE infection, WBC label. Good to differentiate OM from nonunion	in OM, not Charcot
Technesium labeled leukocytes TcHMPAO, Tc exametazime, Ceretec ®	(hexamethylpropyleneamine oxime) for differentiating OM and Charcot WBC isolated from blood sample and re-injected	**in OM, not Charcot

[31] Grayson, M. Lindsay, et al. "Probing to bone in infected pedal ulcers: a clinical sign of underlying osteomyelitis in diabetic patients." Jama 273.9 (1995): 721-723.

[32] Lavery, Lawrence A., et al. "Probe-to-Bone Test for Diagnosing Diabetic Foot Osteomyelitis Reliable or relic?." Diabetes care 30.2 (2007): 270-274.

[33] Shone, Alison, et al. "Probing the validity of the probe-to-bone test in the diagnosis of osteomyelitis of the foot in diabetes." Diabetes Care 29.4 (2006): 945-945.

[34] Thorning, Chandani, et al. "Midfoot and hindfoot bone marrow edema identified by magnetic resonance imaging in feet of subjects with diabetes and neuropathic ulceration is common but of unknown clinical significance." Diabetes care 33.7 (2010): 1602-1603.

Gallium, 67 Citrate	Subacute/CHRONIC, SOFT TISSUE infection. Uptake by WBC, bacterial siderophore, lactoferrin, and iron-binding proteins	**if positive with negative 3rd phase bone scan, r/o OM
Combined Tc & Ga OR Tc & Ind	Tc for bone, Ga for WBC	both positive = OM Ga+ Tc- = cellulitis Ga- Tc+ = charcot
Anti-granulocyte Fab fragment (sulesomab) scan		
PET scan	tracer injected/inhaled to release radioactive positron to produce gamma ray	

TX:

Osteomyelitis cured when:
- no SOI
- stabilized/improved XR findings x 1 year
- sustained healing of wound

Conservative:
- PO or IV antibiotics
  - 6 wks just as good as 12wks (Tone et al, Diabetes care 2015[35])

Surgical:
- s/p amputation, antibiotics for 3-4 weeks OR no antibiotics are both good options
- Amputation
  - Hallux amp: leave 1cm at proximal phalanx
  - Toe amputations: Leave cartilage at MT head as a barrier to infection
  - Partial toe amputations: better than MTPJ disarticulation (prevents toe varus/valgus)
  - Partial 1st ray amp: NOT good for young active patients (transfer lesions)
  - TMA: good functional foot
- **Papineau technique**
  - USE: infected nonunion of long bone
  - Open debridement of bone with cancellous graft
  - No attempt at soft tissue coverage-granulation occurs over graft
  - Superficial bone graft may desiccate and need to remove
  - use split thickness skin graft or wound vac over graft

OM radiographic terms:

1	Osteolysis	Gross bone fragmentation/destruction, radiolucency 10-14 days after onset of symptoms when 30-50% of osseous washout due to inflammatory hyperemia
2	Involucrum	Living bone remodeling around dead bone, CHRONIC OM
3	Cloaca	Tract perforating through opening in involucrum forming sinus/drain, CHRONIC OM
4	Sequestrum	Necrotic, opaque bone fragments separated from living bone by granulation tissue (area of decreased density), *located inside pus*!
	Brodie's abscess	AKA "bone abscess" area of decreased density (lytic) surrounded by dense fibrous tissue/increased sclerotic bone (bone remodeling). Subacute, without purulence or clinical symptoms

---

[35] Tone, Alina, et al. "Six-Week Versus Twelve-Week Antibiotic Therapy for Nonsurgically Treated Diabetic Foot Osteomyelitis: A Multicenter Open-Label Controlled Randomized Study." Diabetes care 38.2 (2015): 302-307.

Garre's sclerosing OM	Type of chronic OM. Nonpurulent, subacute, low-grade, bone appears extremely sclerosed due to marked periosteal bone deposition
Septic arthritis	Subchondral resorption, osteolysis
Rarefaction	Localized decreased bone density
Eburnation	subchondral sclerosis at areas of cartilage loss
Periostitis	Calcification along periosteal surface
Rim sign	in MRI, thin layer of active infection surrounding bone
Other terms	<ul><li>Inc/dec soft tissue density/volume</li><li>Bone/joint destruction<ul><li>Periosteal reaction/periosteal lifting</li><li>Loss of cortical margin</li><li>Sclerosis</li></ul></li></ul>

Chronic osteomyelitis, chronic OM

ET: contiguous spread, present for several weeks
- ability for bacteria to hide in biofilm

TX: PO ABx with bioavailable agents is comparable to IV ABx
- PO: RIFAMPIN +bactrim, fluoroquinolones, linezolid, doxycycline, clindamycin
  for 2-4 months
- Surgical debridement followed by ABx increases cure rate
  - However, no strong evidence for 4-6 wks of therapy s/p surgical debridement

Neurology System

Diabetic neuropathy, peripheral neuropathy, diabetic peripheral neuropathy (DPN)

ET:

Top 3

1) Diabetes
    a. Accumulation of sorbitol/fructose in Schwann cells leading to HYPEROSMOLARITY—>swelling—>cell lysis
    b. Microvascular damage impairs nerve healing
2) Alcoholism
3) Spinal cord disease (lumbar radiculopathy)

- "DANG THE RAPIST"
    o Diabetes, Alcohol (10+ years), Nutrition (vit B12 2/2 metformin/folate), Guillain barre, Tumor, toxins, trauma, thyroid, Hereditary (CMT), Endocrine (thyroid), Radiculopathy, Amyloidosis (deposit of protein in tissues), Polio, Infectious disease (HIV, viral), Sarcoidosis, toxin (lead, mercury)

Differential Diagnosis of Peripheral Neuropathies

Causes	Examples
Metabolic	DM2, hypothyroidism, amyloidosis
Infectious	HIV, Hepatitis, Leprosy
Neoplastic	Carcinoma, myeloma
inflammatory/autoimmune	RA, SLE, Guillain-Barre syndrome
Nutritional deficiences	Alcoholism, vit B12 deficiency, pernicious anemia
Toxicity	Drugs (isoniazid), heavy metals (arsenic, lead), chemotherapy
Hereditary	Charcot-Marie-Tooth, DeJerine Sotta's disease

Nerve injuries

Seddon classification[36]

Neuropraxia	Bruised nerve (occurs in surgery). Damage to myelin, which can regenerate. May lose DTR, mm fcn, vibration, 2 pt discrimination. Repair in days-months	Reversible
Axontmesis	Myelin + axon injury —> Wallerian degeneration Etiology: prolonged compression, ischemia, traction, toxin	Reversible
Neurontmesis	Complete severance Etiology: laceration, gunshot wound, open fracture, puncture	Irreversible

Sunderland classification[37]

class	symptoms

---

[36] Seddon, H. J. "A classification of nerve injuries." British medical journal 2.4260 (1942): 237.
[37] Sunderland, Sydney, and Francis Walshe. "Nerves and nerve injuries." (1968): 9.

class	symptoms
1	neuropraxia
2	axontmesis
3	Disruption of fascicle organization
4	partial severance
5	neurontmesis

DX:
- Light touch: SWMF, ipswich touch test
- Pain: pin prick
- Vibratory
- Reflexes
- SUDOSCAN, QSART
- **NCS/NCV**: velocity of nerve, useful in determining the distribution of nerve lesion.
  - Normal is 40mps
- **EMG**: activity generated by muscle fibers
  - <u>Normal test:</u> amplitude of response proportional to effort
  - <u>Denervation:</u> fasciculations at rest, decreased motor units
- Labs: CBC, Chem7, HgA1C

CP:
1) **Sensory**
   a. <u>Symmetric distal polyneuropathy</u>-MOST COMMON, tingling & numbness in "stocking glove" pattern, loss of protective sensation
   b. <u>Small fiber neuropathy</u>-A delta and C fibers, burning, stabbing, crushing, aching, cramp worse at night
   c. <u>Radicular/Mononeuropathy</u>-cranial and spinal

Spinal tract

Sensation	Spinal tract
Light touch	anterior spinothalamic
Vibration/proprioception	posterior
Pain/temperature	lateral

Nerve Fiber

Nerve fiber	Characteristics
A	Largest myelinated
B	Moderate size, myelinated
C	Small, unmyelinated

2) **Motor**
   a. "Intrinsic minus" atrophy leading to claw toe and hammertoe (extensor substitution), PF 1st MT, cavus foot, DISTAL migration of fat pad towards the toe sulcus
3) **Autonomic (20%)**
   a. Sympathetics and parasympathetics:
      i. GI-gastroparesis (CONSTIPATION), impotence (ED)

23

        ii.   GU-urinary incontinence
        iii. Orthostatic hypotension
        iv. Poor balance/poor gait
        v.   Resting tachycardia
        vi. Anhydrosis, xerosis-dry scaling feet prone to fissuring
        vii. Dishydrotic eczema
        viii. Hyperkeratosis
   b. Reduced capillary flow, LE edema

4) **Neuropathic cachexia:**
   a. weight loss, pain, small fiber neuropathy

TX:
Conservative
- **Capsaicin cream**
  - Burns more at first, depletes substance P, then relieves pain

Surgical:
- Nerve decompression surgery-either common peroneal nerve or tibial nerve

Oral meds

Drug name	Trade name	Dosing rec	Max dose	SE
Gabapentin	Neurontin ®	300 mg	3600mg	Sleepiness
Pregabalin	Lyrica ®	50 mg	100 mg Q3	Swelling
TCA	Amitryptiline			Suicide risk
B12 vitamins	Metanx ®, Nicbid (B3, Niacin)			
Opioid analgesics (tramadol)				
Alpha lipoic acid		600mg		
SSRI/SNRI	Paroxetine, Fluoxetine, sertraline, venlofaxine			
Valproic acid	Valproate			

End Stage renal disease, chronic kidney disease (ESRD/CKD)
CP:
- Uremic myopathy
  - wasting of muscles of foot
- Hemosiderin deposits
  - Found on extensor surface of foot
- Microalbuminuria

Clinical triad:
1) Uremic neuroapthy
   a. due to the accumulation of dialyzable neurotoxins
   b. may overlap with diabetic neuropathy
2) Infection
3) PAD

Charcot Marie Tooth Disease (CMT)
      Hereditary, demyelinating, hypertrophic neuropathy of the peripheral nervous system

ET
- Muscular imbalance of intrinsics and extrinsics

Clinical presentation	Anatomical etiology
Plantarflexed 1st ray	Overpowering of PL over tibialis anterior
Eversion, heel varus	Weakened PB compared to tibialis posterior
Elevation of plantar arch	Fibrosis and shortening of plantar fascia

Cock-up MTPJ and clawing of lesser toes	Recruitment of EHL and EDL as accessory dorsiflexors to balance weakness of TA

EP
- 17-40 per 100,000[38]
- 5x greater in men than women
CP:
- **Autosomal recessive**-present at age 8
- **Autosomal dominant**-present at age 30
- Slow, progressive, slow, distal neuromuscular disease leading to DROP FOOT
    - o Cavus foot (90%)
    - o Equinovarus
- Manifests in first or third decade
- "Stork leg"/"Champagne bottle" legs, due to peroneal atrophy
- Stocking glove neuropathy, decreased DTR, decreased vibratory sensation, decreased proprioception
- Essential tremor
DX: electromyography, molecular analysis
TX:
- Early treatment advised to deal with a more flexible deformity before degenerative changes occur
- Plantar fasciotomy, Jones procedure, DF osteotomy of 1st MT in absence of fixed hindfoot deformity yield best results[39]
- To correct drop foot:
- Conservative
    - o Brace-AFO
    - o Orthotics
- Surgical:
    - o <u>PTT transfer</u>: re-route PTT through interosseus membrane to dorsum of foot
    - o <u>Bridle procedure</u>: (bridle of a horse), re-route PTT through interosseus membrane + anastamosis to 1) tibialis anterior and 2) PL/PB. Avoids varus/valgus deformity of PTT transfer alone.

Friedreich's Ataxia

Hereditary sclerosis of <u>spine</u>
CP:
- Young children to early adolescents, WORSE deformity than CMT

Dropfoot deformity
ET:
- CVA, CMT, multiple sclerorsis, peroneal nerve palsy, brain injury
TX
- stable knee: hinged AFO
- unstable knee (hyperflexion/hyperextension): solid AFO

Charcot neuroarthropathy (CNA), Charcot foot, (neuroarthropathy/neuropathic arthropathy/diabetic neuropathic osteoarthropathy DNOAP)
A destructive, progressive arthropathy due to impaired pain perception and increased blood flow from reflex vasodilaiton
ET:
- Historical origin: TB/syphilis (Tabes Dorsalis)
- <u>3 most common</u>: DM, syringomyelia (spinal cord cyst), tabes dorsalis
- Increased pro-inflammatory cytokines: IL, TNF alpha, RANKL/OPG
- Pathogenesis:
    1) **Autonomic neuropathy** (increased blood flow)
    2) **Motor neuropathy** (muscle imbalance)
    3) **Sensory neuropathy** (patient unaware of microtrauma)
    RF: longstanding DM, high HbA1c values, nephropathy

---

[38] Martyn CN, Hughes RAC. Epidemiology of peripheral neuropathy. J Neurol Neu- rosurg Psychiatry. 1997 Apr;62(4):310-8.

[39] Faldini, Cesare, et al. "Surgical Treatment of Cavus Foot in Charcot-Marie-Tooth Disease: A Review of Twenty-four Cases." The Journal of Bone & Joint Surgery 97.6 (2015): e30.

Theories of Charcot Pathogenesis

Theory	Country	Description
Neurovascular	French, Theory of Charcot	Degeneration of anterior horn of spinal cord (sympathetics/autonomics) —> hypervascular state (reflex vasodilation) —> increased osteoclast activity —> bone resorption
Neurotraumatic	German, Theory of Virchow and Volkmann	Repetitive microtrauma to an insensate foot 2/2 to WB results in unnoticed periarticular fracture and osseous destruction until entire joint is destroyed
RANKL/OPG		overactive osteoclast activity —> bone degeneration
(Neurotrophic)	Original theory	Degeneration of CNS —> decreased bone nutrition

EP:
- Up to 29% in diabetics with peripheral neuropathy or 2/2 any neuropathy
- Men > women
- 30% b/l
  Eichenholtz classification[40] (3 months between each stage)
  o XR findings

Stage	Phase	Description
0 (Prodrome/High-risk Pre-Charcot)	Inflammatory (Charcot in situ)	Warmth, edema, erythema, bounding pulse **Radiograph**: NO CHANGE **MRI**: non-displaced fracture, marrow edema 0-3 months NWB (Charcot still active)
1 (Acute)	Developmental (or fragmentation, destructive)	Increased warmth, edema, erythema **Radiograph**: subchondral bone fragmentation, peri-articular fracture w/ subluxation or dislocation 3-6 months NWB (Charcot still active), or WB in TCC[41]
2	Coalescence	Decreased warmth, edema, erythema **Radiograph**: absorption of osseus debris, new bone formation, fragment coalescence, sclerotic bone ends, ankylosis 6 months-1 year WB okay, (Charcot nonactive)
3	Remodeling / Reconstruction	Resolved warmth, edema, erythema, gross deformity, collapse of longitudinal arch leading to "rocker bottom foot" **Radiograph**: remodeled bone 9 months-1.5 year

RF: age, weight, duration of diabetes, peripheral neuropathy, decreased BMD (osteoporosis)
CP:
- Warm/hot/swollen/dry/painful/red foot or ankle without trauma (>3-4 degrees compared to opposite limb)
  o can be PAINLESS
  o 75% painful even in the presence of neuropathy
- Bounding pulse
- Usually UNILATERAL

[40] Eichenholtz SN. Charcot Joints, p7-8, Springfield, Illinois, Charles C Thomas, 1966
[41] de Souza, Leo J. "Charcot arthropathy and immobilization in a weight-bearing total contact cast." The Journal of Bone & Joint Surgery 90.4 (2008): 754-759.

- Ulceration (40%): Rocker bottom foot (cuboid, navicular, or cuneiform) leading to midfoot ulceration
- Reduced BMD

DX:

Confused with osteomyelitis!
- Bone biopsy gold standard to differentiate difference-Jamshidi needle
- X-ray: REPEAT every 4-6 weeks!!:
  - Atrophic: Subchondral resorption, sclerosis: absent bone plate
    - Bony debris/detritus/destruction OF MULTIPLE BONES (OM only few)
    - Fractures, subluxation/dislocation of TMT joint
    - Abnormal fusion of joints of foot
  - Hypertrophic: joint space narrowing, without osteoporosis
  - **Meary's angle** GREATEST predictor of ulceration (leads to rocker bottom)
  - Reduced CIA
- CT, tech bone scan, MRI
  - Indium 11 bone scane

Anatomic classification (Sanders & Frykberg[42], Brodsky[43], and Schon[44])

Pattern	Sanders and Frykberg	Incidence	Brodsky	Schon
Pattern 1	Forefoot	15%	TMT	TMT
Pattern 2	TMT joint	40%	Peri-talar	NC
Pattern 3	Midfoot: NC/TN/CC joint	30%	A-ankle, B-posterior calcaneus	peri-navicular
Pattern 4	Ankle/STJ	10%	multiple combinations	tarsal
Pattern 5	Calcaneus	5%	Forefoot	

TX:

Lifelong foot care due to recurrent attacks of Charcot deformity and ulceration
1. STOP THE ACUTE (INFLAMMATORY/DEVELOPMENT) PHASE ASAP BY NWB FOR 3-4 MONTHS
2. Serial XR

Conservative-rest, elevation and offload the foot—want to keep foot in a good shape to prevent ulceration
1) Immobilization-reduction of stress
   a. TCC (*in plantigrade position*) non weight bearing to stop the acute inflammatory phase (until erythema/warmth resolves)
      i. Extra padding for bony process (anterior shin, malleoli)
      ii. Caution increased stress on contralateral limb
      iii. RISK: 2X INCREASED HEEL PRESSURE
      iv. Instant TCC: put plaster over a boot—prevents them from taking it off
      v. Immobilize for 4-6 wks, or until <2° temperature difference to contralateral side
2) Transition-decision to transition depends on clinical symptoms—skin lines, edema, XR, temperature
   a. CROW
   b. CAM
   c. Custom molded shoes- maintain stable foot to protect from microtrauma/skin breakdown
      i. AFO
      ii. Bracing
   d. Adjunctive
   e. Bisphosphonates—pamidronate (inconclusive, not approved by FDA)
   f. Bone stimulation

Surgical

[42] Rogers, Lee C., et al. "The Charcot foot in diabetes." Diabetes Care 34.9 (2011): 2123-2129
[43] Brodsky JW. The diabetic foot. In: Coughlin and Mann's 1992 edition
[44] Charcot neuroarthropathy of the foot and ankle. CORR. 1998; 349: 116-131

Goal: stabilize the foot in the best way to prevent ulceration and lost of limb
- Only after bony consolidation
  - o Indications: FOR NON-STABLE, NON BRACEABLE DEFORMITY, recurring ulcer, joint instability, exostosis
- Most Charcot reconstruction surgeries fail 2/2 continued collapse of foot. Always try to surgically position foot in plantigrade position so that when the foot collapses, it will be plantigrade
  - o Create a flat foot without an arch to prevent further collapse
- 6-12 month recovery time and for foot, hardware and bone to stabilize
  - o Long term goal s/p surgery: place patients in motion control shoe
- GOAL: CREATE A PLANTIGRADE FOOT TO NORMALLY DISTRIBUTE PLANTAR PRESSURE
  - o Exostectomy—excision of bones to reduce pressure
  - o Realignment arthrodesis—fusion, using ABx coated nails
  - o ORIF, external fixation (both as good)
  - o TAL or gastroc muscle lengthening to *decrease forefoot* pressure and improve ankle equinus
  - o Amputation
  - o Intramedullary beaming
    - ▯ Midfoot fusion bolt:
      - Medial column (IM screw from talus -->1st MT)
      - Lateral column (between 3rd/4th MT)
    - ▯ supports ligaments
    - ▯ doesn't stress skin (compared to plate)
    - ▯ multiple columns
    - ▯ Risk: IM bone infection, learning curve
  - o Plate-good for isolated medial column

Neuroma, Morton's Neuroma, Joplin's neuroma, perineural fibroma
> *Neuroma: benign fibrotic enlargement of one of the common digital nerves*
> *Perineural fibroma: swelling and growth of tissue surrounding nerves*

Histology: degeneration of myelinated fibers, thickening and hyalinization of epineural/endoneural vv, fibrosis of epineurium and perineurium

ET:
- Mechanical:
  - o Chronic mictrotrauma, nerve compression/entrapment syndrome: DEGENERATION, demyelination, peri-neural fibrosis 2/2 shearing against deep transverse MT ligament (intermetatarsal compression neuritis) or MT head (located dorsal to nerve)
  - o Biomechanical foot type-pronation, hypermobility
- Ischemia

RF: Shoegear (heels, small toebox), forefoot fat pad atrophy, equinus, traumatic nerve injury, cavus (piling of MT heads), enlarged MT head

Name	Location	Nerve
Morton	3rd IM space,	3rd common digital nerve, where medial and lateral plantar nerves meet
Joplin	plantar medial of 1st MTPJ	medial plantar proper digital nerve
Capsulitis	2nd interpsace	

EP: Females 30-60 y.o.
CP:
- Thickening of 3rd interspace feeling like walking on a "wrinkled sock" or "pebble"
- Pain with palpation of interspace
- EASILY CONFUSED WITH CAPSULITIS 2/2 HAMMERTOE
- Capsulitis expect interspace pain with MTPJ ROM
- Intermittent burning/electrical/cramping/Tinel's/numbing in forefoot radiating to digits, worse with weight bearing and barefoot walking
- Numbness on both sides of affected interspace

- Pain relieved by massaging area, removal of shoe gear

DX
- Mulder's sign or "Squeeze test"-silent palpable click with pain in IM space upon compression of MT heads
- Gauthier's test-squeeze MT heads together and DF/PF MT repeatedly to elicit pain
- Sullivan's sign (digital divergence)-splaying of digits upon weight bearing due to metatarsus proximus
- XR
   o Metatarsus proximus leading to Sullivan's sign: no correlation with neuroma pain
- MRI/US (not necessary unless clinically unclear)
- NCV, EMG
- Diagnostic injection

TX:

Conservative:
- MT pad, ECSWT, botulinum toxin, NSAIDs, wider toe box, orthotics, physical therapy, biofreeze gel, contrast soaks
- Injections (dorsally, 45 degrees into IM space)
   o Corticosteroid
   o Sclerotherapy (alcohol ablation): 4% sclerosing (dehydrated) alcohol chemicallly neurolyses the nerve via dehydration, necrosis, precipitation of protoplasm, sclerosis of vascular supply
   o Vitamin B12
   o Phenol

Surgical:

Limited evidence that transposition necessary (Cochrane Review 2004[45])
- Excision of neuroma (dorsal or plantar approach)
   o Most common
   o Transect nerve proximal to MT head (to prevent recurrence), cauterize, transpose proximally
   o Epineural tubularization/epineuroplasty—prevent stump neuroma
   o Complications:
      ▪ STUMP NEUROMA 2/2 not resecting nerve proximal enough, incomplete excision, regeneration
      ▪ Resection of digital artery
      ▪ Hammertoe 2/2 to resection of lumbrical tendon
- Nerve decompression
   o Releasing the deep transverse MT ligament
   o minimally invasive or endoscopic
   o can result in greater neuroma pain
- Revisional neuroma
   o For recurrent neuromas
   o Transecting nerve proximal to MT head, implant into muscle
- Cryogenic neuroablation

Tarsal tunnel syndrome (TTS)

ANATOMY:
- Flexor retinaculum (Laciniate ligament) is formed by fascia cruris and deep transverse fascia
- Medial/posterior: flexor retinaculum (lacinate ligament)
- Anterior: distal tibia (medial malleolus)
- Lateral: calcaneus, talus

ET: tibial nerve compression due to compressed tarsal tunnel beneath flexor retinaculum
- Idiopathic #1 most common
- Trauma #2 most common
   o Recurrent ankle sprains
- Overuse-dancers, athletes, runners
- Biomechanical (Functional)
   o Overpronation (STRETCHES tibial N)
      ▪ tightens flexor retinaculum over nerve
   o Cavus (COMPRESSES tibial N)
- Space-occupying lesions
   o Varicosities, ganglion, lipoma, neurilemoma, idiopathic edema, osteophyte
- Anatomical

---

[45] Thomson, Colin E., J. N. Gibson, and Denis Martin. "Interventions for the treatment of Morton's neuroma." The Cochrane Library (2004).

- o   If tibial N bifurcates into medial/lateral plantar N early
- o   If medial calcaneal N comes off lateral plantar N (normally comes off medial plantar N)
- • Inflammatory conditions
  - o   RA, tendonitis, synovitis

CP:
- UNILATERAL pain, parasthesia, numbness, tingling, burning, abnormal sensation in **medial hindfoot and plantar foot**
- Discomfort worsened with standing, relieved with shoe removal

DX:
- Valleix's sign-**proximal** radiation of tibial nerve
- Tinel's sign-**distal** radiation of pain
- Pinprick and two-point discrimination test
- Phalen's maneuver-PF and inversion of foot to reproduce symptoms
- DF eversion test/FF abduction maneuver-abduct the foot to reproduce symptoms
- Turk's test aka Perthe's tourniquet test-r/o venous etiology
- EMG/NCS-prolonged motor conduction velocity/prolonged distal motor latency
  - o   can be negative
  - o   check at 1st dorsal interossei
- Pressure sensitive sensory device (PSSD): measures cutaneous pressure threshold
  - • US/MRI

DDX: Make sure to r/o:
- Radiculopathy: positive straight leg test, calf mm atrophy
- Sensory polyneuropathy: b/l presentation, stocking glove sensory loss

TX:
- Conservative
  - o   NSAIDs, steroid injection, orthoses (heel lift, medial heel wedge), compression stockings
- Surgical
  - o   Tarsal tunnel release: 1) Release flexor retinaculum 2) release abductor fascia 3) release plantar branches of posterior tibial nerve
    - ▪ **Low success rate in those without space occupying lesions**
  - o   Barrier technique-to prevent scar tissue formation of nerve
    - ▪ Silicone entubulation
    - ▪ Saphenous vein graft wrapping

Baxter's neuritis
ET:
- Entrapment of the first branch of lateral calcaneal nerve
- Misdiagnosed as plantar fasciitis

DX:
- Elicit Tinel's sign

CP: pain AFTER activity (plantar fasciitis is first step pain)

TX:
- Surgical:
  - o   Neurolysis-procedure of choice
  - o   Remove a portion of superficial/deep fascia of abductor hallucis, plantar fascia, and heel spur (if present)

Lumbar radiculopathy (Sciatica)
ET: compressed/herniated disk, compression of the nerve root
CP:
- Straight leg raise-back pain
- Foot numbness-depending on which spinal levels are affected

Multiple sclerosis
ET:
- Autoimmune chronic inflammatory disease leading to demyelination of CNS
- Disease of UMN only
CP:
- Motor, sensory, cerebellar, visual attacks-optic neuritis, blindness, bladder dysfunction
- Charcot's triad: nyastagmus, tremor, scanning speech

- Hyperactive LE reflexes
- Exacerbated by heat

Amyotrophic lateral sclerosis (Lou Gehrig's disease)
ET: Disease of UMN and LMN
CP: **HYPER-REFLEXIA** wasting, weakness, cramps, twitching, spasticity, slurred speech, increased DTR

Guillain barre syndrome, Landry's paralysis
ET: precipitated by infection
CP: drop foot, symmetrical muscle weakness, decreased DTR, death via respiratory paralysis

Complex regional pain syndrome (CRPS), reflex sympathetic dystrophy (RSD), Sudek's atrophy, causalgia
- CRPS I (AKA RSD): **without definable nerve** disorder, bone/joint/muscle pain. Sympathetic overactivity
- CRPS II (AKA causalgia): **with definable nerve** that has been damaged, burning pain
  ET: UNKNOWN, psychogenic,
- CRPS I: injury, immobilization
- CRPS II: precipitating trauma, crush injury, fracture, ankle sprain
  RF: female, >40yo, PMHx anxiety and depression
  NH:

Stages of CRPS I (RSD)- "red, white & blue"

	Symptoms	Timing
Acute stage (RED)	Pain, edema, erythema	Days-weeks
Dystrophic stage (WHITE)	Motor changes develop	3-6 months
Atrophic stage (BLUE)	Decreased pain, atrophic, waxy	>6 months

CP:
- Pain NOT at surgical site
- **Hyperalgesia:** (pain out of proportion), burning pain
- **Allodynia:** (pain developing from non painful stimuli)
- **Dystonia:** sustained muscle contraction causing twisting, repetitive movements, and abnormal posture. Rigid, reluctant to move joints
- **Dysesthesia:** "unpleasant" sensation to touch
- Autonomic disturbance/trophic (nerve) changes
  - Smooth, red, shiny skin, hair changes, osteopenia, altered skin blood flow
- Motor changes: loss of function, tremor, dystonia
- Skin changes: bullae, ulcer, edema
- Pain as a TRIGGER
- Psychological-depression, anxiety
DX:
- CLINICAL DIAGNOSIS
- Imaging: non sensitive/specific
  - XR-**Sudek's atrophy**-osteopenia
  - Bone scan
- Thermography
  - DECREASED temperature, possibly increased temperature around joints
- Blunt pressure testing, brush evoked pain test, pain mapping
- Tourniquet ischemia test to diminish allodynia-painful
- QSART (quantitative sudomotor axon reflex test)-more for research purpose
- Diagnostic nerve block
TX:
- CATCH EARLIER (2wks)
  - begin neurological stimulation. DO NOT immobilize
- Medications:
  - Vitamin C as prophylaxis

- o Gabapentin-clonidine-ketamine gel
- o Corticosteroids (best earlier when inflammation present)
- o Opioids
- o NMDA receptor antagonists
- PT/OT
- Neurological:
  - o Spinal cord stimulation (SCS)
  - o Transcutaneous electrical nerve stimulation (TENS)
    - ▪ mild electrical current to block pain message
- Do NOT use cold/immobilization, regional blockade

Vascular System

PAD, PVD (peripheral arterial disease, peripheral vascular disease)
ET: Atherosclerosis
EP: Hispanics and African Americans
NH:
- Intermittent claudication —> rest pain —> gangrene
- Occlusion distal to trifurcation
- Can progress into critical limb ischemia
RF:
- #1 diabetes
  - o More asymptomatic in DM pts 2/2 neuropathy
  - o present later in life, greater risk amputation
  - o perform ABI in DM >50 y.o.
- #2 smoking
  - o Age, obesity, sedentary lifestyle, high cholesterol, high blood pressure, family history
CP:
- Rest pain relieved with DEPENDENCY
- *Ischemic pain: mimicking ingrown toenail*
- Most sensitive: 1) absent pulses 2) femoral bruit 3) cool skin
- Hair loss, smooth and shiny skin, pallor, cyanosis, dusky gray appearance of skin
- Elevation dependency test: dependent RUBOR (don't confuse with cellulitis!), PALLOR with elevation
- Numbness, hyporeflexia
- Muscle atrophy
- Life-threatening risks: MI, stroke
DX:
XR:
- **Monckeberg's sclerosis**-calcification in the tunica media
- Medial (calcific) sclerosis (Monckeberg's sclerosis—tubular, serpiginous calcification)
Noninvasive testing:
- Indications: nonhealing wound >4 wks, gangrenous changes, cyanosis, rest pain, absent pulses
Overview of Vascular Imaging

Modality	Description	Benefits	Limitations
Continuous wave doppler	transmits and receives sound waves to evaluate rate of blood flow in vv	fast, non-invasive, cost-effective	technician and body habitus dependent. Cannot localize location of obstruction
ABI (segmental pressure)	ratio of blood pressure between brachial and ankle arteries	fast, non-invasive, cost-effective	can be falsely elevated 2/2 arterial calcinosis in DM and renal dz

Modality	Description	Benefits	Limitations
TBI (toe brachial pressure)	Ratio of BP between brachial and toe arteries	Superior to ABI in patiens with arterial calcification. TBI >0.7 can r/o PAD	
Segmental pressure volume	BP cuffs placed at several intervals on legs	For patients with poorly compressible vv	
Skin perfusion pressure (SPP)	Laser doppler measurement that uses BP cuff at ankle	Measure of cutaneous capillary circulation, more sensitive	Requires specialized equipment
Plethysmography/pulse volume recordings (PVR)	changes in volume, air, or blood flow as well as arterial pulsatility	fast, non-invasive, cost-effective	usually combined with ABI
TcPO2	local tissue perfusion and skin oxygenation using local electrodes on skin	fast, non-invasive, cost-effective	limitation in accuracy 2/2 edema, skin temperature, inflammation, pharmacological agents
Ultrasound, duplex ultrasound	sonography to visualize vv cailber, obstruction, flow, and characterize plaque lesions	fast, non-invasive, cost-effective	technician and body habitus dependent. difficult assessing distal and smaller vv
CT angiography (CTA)	cross-sectional imaging providing 360 degree reconstruction of vv	Faster than MRA, non invasive, cheaper than traditional angiography, better spatial resolution	contrast nephrotoxicity, imaging obscured by vv calcification
MR angiography (MRA)	cross-sectional imaging providing 360 degree reconstruction of vv	Non-invasive, no obstruction of vv calcifcation evident in CT angiogrpahy	lengthy exam, expensive, gadolinium nephrotoxicity (dehydration, CHF, >70yo, DM, concurrent nephrotoxic drug), image obscured by venous artifact, limited spatial resolution
Conventional angiography, digital subtraction angiography	inject radiopaque contrast agent into blood vv and imaging using XR	GOLD STANDARD, esp during evaluation fo distribution of PVD when planning revascularization. can also use CO_2 to create radiographic contrast, less nephrotoxic. Simultaneous endovascular intervention	Invasive, caution renal impairment 2/2 contrast
SPY-real time angiography	injection of dye and monitor under	live, intraoperative capabilities	

ABI (ankle brachial index) or AAI (ankle arm index) or TBI (toe brachial index)

- Pick the higher systolic value of DP vs PT divided by highest systolic arm pressure
- 1) measure at rest 2) treadmill until claudication symptoms and re-measure 3) if ABI drops 15-20%, diagnostic of PAD
- TBI: UNAFFECTED by tunica media calcifications
  - o >0.75 Normal, <0.25 Severe.

ABI	Interpretation
>1.3	Calcified
0.9-1.3	Normal
0.6-0.9	Mild obstruction
0.4-0.6	Moderate obstruction
<0.4	Severe obstruction

TcPO2 (transcutaneous oxygen pressure) aka transcutaneous oxygen monitoring (TCOM)
- a measurement of microvasculature
- **>30mmHg is predictive of healing potential**
- CONS: edema, skin temperature, inflammation, pharmacologic can skew results

TcPO2	Interpretation
>55mmHg	Healing
45-55mmHg	Uncertain
<30-40mmHg	No healing

Doppler ultrasound, Color doppler ultrasound, duplex ultrasound
- Grayscale or color flow
  - o <u>Normal</u> = bi/triphasic sharp, HIGH pitched. (Second sound is backward flow)
  - o <u>Abnormal</u> = monophasic, swishing, LOW pitched
- Good after re-vascularization, not for microvascular disease
  - o for perforating peroneal A, block lateral malleolar branch from anterior tibial A

TX:
- <u>Compression stockings</u>
  - o TED (thombo-embolic deterrent) hose
  - o Custom compression stockings 15-60 mmHg
    - ▪ 15: DVT prophylaxis
    - ▪ 25-35: venous insufficiency
    - ▪ 40-50: lymphedema
  - o Contra: non-ambulatory, severe arterial insufficiency
- <u>Revascularization</u>
  - o GOAL: restore direct, pulsatile flow to the foot
  - o 2 types of repair:
    - ▪ **Endovascular repair**-with/without stenting
    - ▪ **Open repair**-bypass, artherectomy
  - o Surgical intervention 3 days s/p bypass resulted in maximum TcPO2 levels[46]
  - o **Angiosomes**-anatomic region that specific artery supplies. Preferably revascularize the artery that supplies the ischemic region of interest
  - o Auto-amputation, prevent infection, leave stable eschar

PAD Medication

---

[46] Arroyo CI, Tritto VG, Buchbinder D, et al. Optimal waiting period for foot salvage surgery following limb revascularization. J Foot Ankle Surg. 2002;41(4):228-32.

	Trade name	Dosage	Effect
Aspirin		325mg QD	
Clopidogrel	Plavix ®	75mg QD	tx for ACS
Pentoxyfylline	Trental ®	400mg TID	reduce leg pain/cramps, inc RBC flexibility
Cilostazol	Pletal		same as Trental. vasodilation
Enoxaparin	Lovenox		
Fondaparinux	Arixtra		
Dabigatran	Pradaxa		

Anticoagulants

Drug	Dose	Use
Heparin	5,000-10,000 units	DVT prophylaxis
Warfarin (Coumadin ®)	10mg PO QD	DVT prophylaxis
Streptokinase/Urokinase/TPA (alteplace)	TPA = tissue plasminogen activator, shortest half life	**Thrombolytic agent**-converts plasminogen —> plasmin to dissolve clot. Risk STROKE

Critical limb ischemia (CLI), arterial embolism, dry gangrene, wet gangrene,

ET:
- Originally used to describe ischemia in patients WITHOUT diabetes
- Arterial embolism, emoblic event

NH:
- Intermittent claudication—pain worst after walking ___# blocks, (need to rest for 15 minutes because of the pain). Pain relieved with rest
- Rest pain: pain relieved with dependent position, worst at night. If relieved with activity —> VENOUS problem
- Gangrene: 40% of CLI patients without revascularization will experience a major amputation within 1 year

CP:
- **Ischemic rest pain**—severe pain while person is not moving, non-healing sores, pain/numbness, shiny/smooth/dry skin, thickened nails
- Coldness/numbness in toes

Type	Blood loss	Bacterial infection
Dry	gradual	NO
Wet	sudden (burns, freezing, emoblism)	YES, likely —> sepsis

TX:
- Revascularization via vascular surgery

WIFi classification sytem[47]: "Wound, Infection, Foot infection"
- Use for patients with ischemic rest pain

---

[47] Mills, Joseph L., et al. "The Society for Vascular Surgery lower extremity threatened limb classification system: risk stratification based on Wound, Ischemia, and foot Infection (WIfI)." Journal of vascular surgery 59.1 (2014): 220-234.

Wound:

Grade	Ulcer	Gangrene	Clinical description
0	Ischemic rest pain with no ulcer	No gangrene	No wound
1	Ulcer with no exposed bone	No gangrene	Salvageable with digital amputation
2	Ulcer with exposed bone, joint, tendon, heel wound without calcaneal involvement	Gangrenous changes limited to digits	Digital amputations >3, or TMA
3	Ulcer with forefoot/midfoot, heel wound with calcaneal involvement	Extensive gangrene to forefoot/Midfoot, heel necrosis	Salvageable only with complex reconstruction, Chopart/Lisfranc amputation

Ischemia:

Grade	ABI	Ankle systolic pressure	TcPO2
0	>0.80	>100mmHg	>60mmHg
1	0.6-0.79	70-100mmHg	40-59mmHg
2	0.4-0.59	50-70mmHg	30-39mmHg
3	<0.39	<50mmHg	<40mmHg

Varicose vein, sunburst varices, spider veins

ET: valvular incompetence causes superficial vein dilation. Usually great saphenous
RF: standing, heavy lifting, pregnancy
EP: female >>males
CP: itching, asymptomatic, cramps relieved with elevation, edema, telangiectasia
Sunburst varices/spider veins-subcutaneous varicose veins, purple color
TX: elastic stockings, elevation, exercise, surgical excision

Superficial Thrombophlebitis

ET: inflammation of superficial vein due to history of recent trauma or IV, DVT.
CP: palpable linear cord, erythema, warmth, similar to DVT
TX: self-resolving in 1-2 weeks

Venous stasis ulcer, chronic venous insufficiency, venous insufficiency, post phlebitic syndrome, post thrombotic syndrome
Usually superficial vein incompetence (great or lesser saph)

ET:
- Deep venous thrombophlebitis 2/2 **valvular incompetency** leading to reversal flow of venous blood from DEEP —> SUPERFICIAL.
- Venous hypertension (increase in superficial venous pressure) 2/2 to venous reflux leading to ulceration
- Venous regurgitation-transudation of inflammatory mediators into the subcutaneous tissue
- Iliocaval venous obstruction (IVCO) aka May-Thurner syndrome
  - compression of the iliac vein against vertebrae or aortic bifurcation
  - greater risk in females
  - risk for DVT and DVR (reflux)

RF: age > 80 y.o.
CP:
- Rest pain RELIEVED with ELEVATION or activity
- Lipodermatosclerosis (LDS)
  - Hyperpigmentation (hemosiderin deposits) due to leaked RBC from venous HTN
  - Thin, shiny, atrophic, cyanotic, pitting edema, erythema, induration, scaling, fibrosis, dermatitis
- Inflammation of fat (panniculitis)
- "Gaiter distribution" or "inverted champagne bottle"—constricting band circumferentially around ankle
- Pruritis 2/2 to eczemoid weeping dermatitis
- Varicosities
- **Ulcerations** ABOVE medial malleolus
- **Post-phlebitic syndrome** aka **post-thrombotic syndrome (PTS)**
  - Similar symptoms to DVT

DX:

- Trendelenburg test-elevate leg to empty veins, tourniquet to occlude superficial veins. Have patient stand. If veins fill rapidly, venous system incompetent.
- Perthe's tourniquet test aka Turk's test-BP cuff on elevated thigh to cut off superficial veins. Patient will walk to evaluate deep veins
  - **Incompetent deep valve**: blood will move from deep to superficial veins
- CT or MR venography
- Duplex ultrasound

NH:
- Long term varicose ulcer progress into SCC

TX:
- Compression therapy (35-40mmHg):
  - Contraindicated in PAD (ABI < 0.8), hx DVT
  - Pneumatic compression devices, TED (thombo-embolic deterrent) hose, compression stockings
- Bandage:
  - Rigid (Unna boot)
  - Elastic (ACE, compression stocking)
  - Multilayer (**Profore** ®)-the best, add an ELASTIC layer to rigid layer
- Wound care: Resolution of edema is necessary for wound healing!
  - **Unna boot**-impregnated with zinc oxide and calamine
    - "foldback overlap" across the tibial crest
    - Kerlix
    - ACE bandage (make sure to unravel first), then wrap loosely around leg, able to se the wrinkles in the bandage.
- **Wet to dry dressings** with normal saline, followed by corticosteroids (0.5% hydrocortisone cream)
- Burow's solution (aluminum acetate, antibacterial)
- Elevation
- Oral meds
  - LMWH, pentoxyfylline (Trental ®), subcut warfarin, aspirin
  - Long term: oral warfarin (Coumadin) maintain INR 1.5-2
- Surgery
  - Does NOT improve ulcer healing but reduces recurrence

DVT (deep venous thrombosis), venous thromboembolism disease (VTED), pulmonary embolism (PE)
partial or complete oclusion of vein by thrombus with inflammatory reaction

ET:

Virchow's triad:
1) Venous stasis-arrhythmias, A-fib, MI, CHF, immobilization, obesity, stroke, tobacco
2) Hypercoagulability-malignancy, oral contraceptives, surgery, polycythemia, factor 5 Leiden deficiency, protein C&S deficiency, oral contraceptives, infection
3) Endothelial injury-trauma, fracture

Pulmonary embolism: blockage of one or more of pulmonary arteries by a thrombus that has travelled from another part of the body via deep venous system

Table 1

Risk factors for venous thromboembolism disease during management of foot and ankle conditions

Patient Specific	Treatment Specific	Surgery/Injury Specific
Primary		
Personal history of VTED	Immobilization >4 wk	
Hypercoagulability		
Active/recent (<6 mo) cancer		
Secondary		
Advanced age (>60)	Non-weightbearing	Achilles tendon rupture
Obesity (BMI >30)	Hospitalization	Ankle fracture
Family history of VTED	Bed rest	Total ankle replacement
OCP or HRT use		Hindfoot arthrodesis
Varicose veins		General anesthesia
Diabetes mellitus or >1 comorbidity		
Severe foot/ankle injury		

RF:
- #1 risk factor is history of previous DVT
- Well's criteria

CP: red, hot, indurated, pain relieved with elevation, worsened with dependency, edema, erythema, tenderness
- 25% —> pulmonary embolism (triad: hemopytsis, SOB, chest pain)
- DX PE: VQ scan, CT angiography
- Absence of pain IF patency of superficial vv

EP:
- 300,000-600,000 new diagnoses each year, >60,000 deaths each year in U.S.
- 0.05%-28% of patients s/p surgery distal to knee
- 20%-30% mortality with PE

DX:

Clinical:
- Homan's sign-calf pain with DF
- Pratt's test-squeezing proximal calf (popliteal V) to elicit pain
- Bancroft's sign-calf pain with palpation against tibia

Labs:
- D dimer: >500 -fibrin fragment linked to fibrin degradation. Indicates thrombotic disease

Imaging:
- Duplex Doppler venous ultrasound
  - examines deep and superficial veins
  - more accurate for veins below knee, but less invasive
- Contrast venography
  - GOLD STANDARD, but invasive.
  - Can differentiate between old and new DVT

TX:

Prophylaxis:
- Reduce risk factors
- Routine chemical prophylaxis is NOT WARRANTED for foot and ankle surgery requiring ankle immobilization[48]
- Mechanical prophylaxis
- Early mobilization

Acute:
- IV unfractioned heparin: Law of 8018: 80mg/kg bolus, then 18mg/kg/hr

---

[48] Fleischer, Adam E., et al. "American College of Foot and Ankle Surgeons' Clinical Consensus Statement: Risk, Prevention, and Diagnosis of Venous Thromboembolism Disease in Foot and Ankle Surgery and Injuries Requiring Immobilization." The Journal of Foot and Ankle Surgery (2015).

- LMWH (Lovenox): 1mg/kg Q12

Chronic:
- Warfarin (coumadin)
- Consider IVC filter (insert in IVC inferior to renal vv)

Pitting edema scale

Stage	Depth	Disappears
1+	2mm	Rapid
2+	4mm	10-15 seconds
3+	6mm	60 seconds
4+	8mm	2-5 minutes

Thromboangiitis Obliterans (Buerger's Disease)

small/medium vv vasculitis

ET: hypersensitivity to smoking

Raynaud's phenomenon

ET: cold or stress causing paroxysmal vasospasm of digits

Lymphedema

Accumulation of excessive lymph fluid

ET: obstruction or destruction of lymphatics
CP: <u>Nonpitting edema</u>, chills, fever, red hot swollen leg, tender lymph nodes

Lymphagitis

Inflammation of lymphatics

ET: Bacterial infection
CP: painful red streaks along the course of the vessel, palpable painful lymph nodes, fever, chills with portal of entry

Lymphadenitis

inflammation of lymph nodes due to infection

Elephantiasis

ET: mosquitoes causing filariasis (lymphatic obstruction)
CP: chronic LE edema, venous insufficiency ulcer

Dermatology System

Dry Skin (Xerosis)

TX:
- Keratolytics
  - Urea cream for hyperkeratotic skin
  - Salicyclic acid
  - Ammonim lactate (Amlactin ®)

Tinea pedis (Athlete's foot), pustular tinea pedis

ET:
- T rubrum (60%), T mentagrophytes (20%), E floccosum
  - fungus produces keratinase that destroys stratum corneum at moderate pH

CP:

- Dry, xerotic, scaly skin, in conjunction with onychomycosis
- interdigital maceration
- 85% of people are RESISTANT
- **Pustular tinea pedis**: pustule formation at plantar medial arch

DX:
- scrape off border for KOH stain

TX: KOH prep BEFORE starting antifungals

Dressings
- **Burow's solution**-aluminum acetate wet dressings

Topical creams
- **Antifungals**
    - AZOLEs: 1% Clotrimazole, Ketoconazole
    - terbinafine or naftifine BETTER than azoles[49] (Cochrane 2007)
- **Steroids**-1% hydrocortisone
- Castellani paint—topical fungicide with phenol

Oral:
- **Lamisil** (terbinafine) 250mg x 90 days, **itraconazole, fluconazole, griseofulvin** (less effective)
    - terbinafine = itraconazole[50] (Cochrane 2012)
    - terbinafine > griseofulvin
- Vinegar (UCLA dermatologist)-to decrease pH so the fungal keratinase cannot function

Hemorrhagic cellulitis
ET: brown recluse spider, TNF alpha
CP: non blanchable erythema, bullae
TX: prednisone

Lichen Simplex Chronicus
CP: Self-perpetuating chronic itching and scratching —> thick, leathery brown skin

Livedo reticularis
CP: lace-like mottled vascular venous pattern 2/2 to edema and swelling of veins

Pernio
ET: inflammatory lymphocytic vasculitis 2/2 degradation by neutrophils
RF: cold exposure
CP: pruritic and/or painful erythematous violaceous acral lesions
TX: Systemic corticosteroids, low-dose nifedipine, avoid cold temperature

Scabies
ET: Sarcoptes scabiei, severe itching
CP: hands, penis. Find the bug in the pustule

Erythema multiforme
ET: herpes, sulfa drugs
CP: multiple patches of erythema

Ecthyma
ET: usually S Aureus, strep pyogenes
CP: superficial infection into dermis, crust erosions, ulcers

Lichen aureus
ET: form of progressive pigmented purpura
CP: orange rust colored coin shaped patch

Mycosis fungoides

---

[49] Crawford F, Hollis S "Topical treatments for fungal infections of the skin and nails of the foot." The Cochrane Library 2007
[50] Bell-Syer, Sally EM, et al. "Oral treatments for fungal infections of the skin of the foot." The Cochrane Library (2012)

ET: cutaneous T-cell lymphoma
CP: presents as erythematous eczematoid or psoriasis-form plaque/tumor

Keratotic lesions (heloma molle, heloma durum, intractable plantar keratosis (IPK)
CP: painful lesion under WB portion of foot, usually MT head
- Heloma molle-interdigial abutting of condyles
- Heloma durum-dorsal IPJ or lateral 5th IPJ
    o   Linear-FF valgus
    o   Distal and lateral to MT head-overpronation
NH: Mechanical stress —> keratotic lesion grows —> inflammation
RF: Cavus foot, flatfoot, hammertoes, wide/splaying foot, hallux valgus, bunionette, ill-fitting shoe gear
TX: padding, offloading

Infantile digital inclusion body fibromatosis
CP: pediatric painless, firm nodule in the toes, multi-centric

Porokeratosis plantaris discreta (Steinberg's lesion), porotype lesion, porokeratoma
ET: plantar pressure, sweat pore obstruction
CP:
1)   hyperkeratotic tissue with crater-like *central nucleated core with white or yellow-white* appearance.
2)   tenderness with side to side compression of the lesion
TX: debridement, offloading, salicyclic acid, cryosurgery

Cutaneous horn (cornu cutaneum)

Plantar wart, plantar verrucae
ET: viral (HPV) infection
CP: No skin lines, peppered appearance, pinpoint hemosiderin deposits
TX:
- DEBRIDE TO BLEEDING POINT:
- Spontaneous remission in 60%
- Cryotherapy (liquid nitrogen)
    o   mainstay of treatment, @ 2 and 4 week intervals
    o   freezing destroys cells that harbor virus
- Phenol
- Retinoids-adapalene (same chemical as acne treatment)[51]
- Salicyclic acid
- Acetic acids
- Cantharone (Cantharidin) every 2 weeks x4 applications. Requires occlusion for up to 24 hrs.
- Electricodesiccation & curettage-can leave scar, requires local anesthetic
- CO_2 laser-can be difficult
- Surgical excision
- Podophyllun-antimitotic agent
- Imiquimod-cause patient's body to produce interferon
- Bleomycin-injection can cause tissue necrosis
- 5-fluorouracil-pyrimidine analogue that inhibits DNA synthesis

Verrucous carcinoma
CP: WB surface of foot, in chronic non-healing wounds, slow growing, burrowing pattern, possible malodorous drainage
DX: Biopsy with histological analysis by pathology
TX: Wide excision with tumor-free margins

Proteus syndrome
ET: localized redundant/hypertrophic skin with underlying bone hypertrophy
CP: associated with lipomas, epidermal nevi, vascular lesions, clotting disorders

---

[51] Gupta R, Gupta S. Topical adapalene in the treatment of plantar warts; randomized comparative open trial in comparison with cryotherapy. Indian J Dermatol. 2015; 60(1):102.

Pyogenic granuloma, capillary hemangioma
- Benign vascular lesion, solitary glistening red papules, easily bleed

Epithelioma cuniculatum
- A form of well-differentiated squamous cell carcinoma

Marjolin ulcer
Chronic no healing ulcer 2/2 to:
- malignancy (squamous cell carcinoma)
- previous burn injury
- OM sinus tract

Molluscum contagiosum
- Pearly umbilicated popular epithelial lesions containing numerous inclusion bodies
- Viral infection of skin

Dermatofibrosarcoma protueberans (DFSP)
ET: form of low grade fibrosarcoma
CP: "tuber" formation, like a potato, may metastasize to regional lymph nodes. Locally aggressive with high recurrence rate after excision

Interdigital maceration
Erythrasma vs tinea pedis vs heloma molle
Wood's lamp

Color	Organism	Disease	Clinical present	Treatment
Coral red	Corynebacterium minutissimum	Erythrasma	red, brown, scaly, macerated, itchy	Erythromycin drops
Green	Pseudomonas			Ciprofloxacin drops
Yellow	tinea versicolor			

Merkel cell carcinoma
ET: form of high-grade neuroendocrine carcinoma
CP: rapidly proflierates and exhibits early metastasis. 50% have metastasized att time of diagnosis
TX: requires sentinel lymph node biopsy

Renal cell carcinoma
ET: one of the most common carcinomas to metastasize to the feet
CP: notoroious for late metastases

Malignant melanoma
CP:
- Diameter >6mm (pencil eraser size)
- Hutchinson's sign: 1) pigmentation of proximal nail fold indicative of subungual melanoma OR Bowen's disease (benign) 2) vesicles on the tip of the nose associated with herpes zoster

Type of melanoma	Details
Superficial spreading	Most common, spreads wide before deep
Nodular	WORST prognosis, ulceration, colorful
Lentigo	SLOW, elderly, least metastasis
Acral	Melanotic whitlow—located on palms, soles, Hutchinson's sign, African American

Clarks levels

1	Epidermis
2	Basement membrane
3	Papillary dermis
4	Reticular dermis
5	Subcutaneous tissue

Breslow's (in mm)

1	<0.75
2	0.75-1.5
3	1.5-4
4	> 4

Pyoderma gangrenosum

ET:
- Pathergy-minor trauma leads to development of skin lesions/ulcers resistant to healing, most commonly in LE
- Associated with inflammatory disorders (50%) (UC, Crohn's, IBS, inflammatory arthropathy, RA, hematological disorder)
- Paraneoplastic phenomenon
- Neutrophilic ulcerating skin disease

EP:
- Rare- 3-10 per million

CP:
- 1 or multiple wounds
- very PAINFUL
- "Cat's paw" appearance
- "Cigarette paper" atrophic scars
- small papule —> large ulcers with dusky red/erythematous, undermining/**purple "violaceous" raised overhanging edges**
- hypergranular, necrotic base
- systemic symptoms-myalgia, arthralgia, malaise, fever

DDX: venous ulceration, vasculitis, infection, necrobiosis lipoidica,

DX:
- **A diagnosis of exclusion**
- Obtain <u>punch biopsy</u>-ulcer border and adjacent skin
- rule out infectious etiology which may mimic PG
- Colonoscopy to rule out GI symptoms

TX:

Surgery:
- Poor response to debridement and skin graft—PG may start at skin graft site

Medications: REDUCE INFLAMMATION
- "triple cream"-nyastatin, bactroban, steroid
- topical-tacrolimus, aczone
- intralesional-triamcinolone, cyclosporine
- IVIG
- Steroids
- aggressive immunosuppression
- Biologics-etanercept, infliximab,

Cutaneous manifestation of diabetes

Necrobiosis lipoidica diabeticorum	Red, flat well circumscribed lesions on shin with waxy, yellow center ET: diabetic microangiopathy inflammatory 2/2 collagen degeneration granulomatous response-deposition of glycoprotein, immunoglobulin in blood vv trauma DX: skin biopsy-NECROBIOSIS TX: no treatment
Xanthoma diabeticorum	Yellow papules over extensor surfaces
Bullous diabeticorum	Clear fluid blisters
Diabetic dermopathy	Atrophic hyperpigmented, hemosiderin deposits, circumscribed skin lesions

Frostbite

ET: cellular damage due to jagged ice crystals and ischemia
TX: if tissue might be re-frozen, do NOT thaw. Re-freezing increases tissue necrosis
CP: firm, hard, cool to touch, waxy white, blotchy blue-gray
- edema, hemorrhagic blister, necrosis, gangrene may occur

Degree	Description
1	peeling
2	blistering
3	skin death, hemorrhagic blister, SC involvement
4	full thickness freezing, loss of limb

TX:
- constant warmth with gentle pressure

Burns

TX: leave intact blisters alone, unless restricting blood flow
Total Body Surface Area (Rule of 9's)

Body part	%
each leg	18
each arm	9
total front and back chest	36
head	9

Degrees of Burns

	Description	Thickness	Sensation
1st Degree	sunburn, to papillary dermis, no bullae	Partial	yes

	Description	Thickness	Sensation
2nd Degree	deeper dermis, bullae,	Partial	yes
3rd Degre	subcutaneous fat, painless, charred	Full	possibly
4th Degree	exposed tendon/bone	Full	no

Madura foot, eumycetoma

	Fungal (eumycetoma)	Bacterial (actinomycetoma)
Prevalance	40%	60%
Species	Pseudallescheria boydii (Scedosporium apiospermum), Madurella mycetomatis.	Actinomadura madurae, actinomadura pelletieri, nocardia species, Streptomyces somaliensis
Treatment	Ketoconazole, itraconazole, amphotercin	Bactrim, rifampin, dapsone, streptomycin
Prognosis	Worse, may need surgery as definitive treatment	Better response to antibiotics

ET: local trauma-cut that enters fascial planes, eventually involving bone
EP: most cases in the "Madura belt" in Africa (Sudan) and India
CP: painless swelling, discharge, usually presents at an advanced stage, sinus tract formation with sulfur granules
DX: XR, MRI, microscopy and culture of exudate, skin and bone biopsy
TX: medical management, surgery-especially when bone involved

Nail Pathology

- **Mee's lines**-transverse white band (arsenic poisoning)
- **Beau's lines**-horizontal depression due to transient arrest of nail growth. (stress, MI, PE, fever, trauma)
- **Koilonychia**-spoon nail (iron deficiency anemia)
- **Muehrcke's nail**-transverse white band, nephrotic syndrome
- **Onychauxic**-thickening of nail
- **Eponychium**-cuticle (proximal nail fold)
- **Hyponychium**-distal nail fold
- **Hutchinson's sign**-1) pigmentation of proximal nail fold indicative of subungual melanoma OR Bowen's disease (benign)

Ingrown toenail, onychocryptosis
ET/RF:
- Improper nail trimming "bathroom surgery"
- Athletes
- Biomechanical-hypermobile first ray, pronation, subungual exostosis
- Poorly fitted shoes
- Pediatrics secondary from nail sucking
- Immune compromised

EP: Young males, hallux nails
CP:
- PARONYCHIA-local infection 2/2 to ingrown nail
- Pain worse in shoes, erythema, edema, foul odor, "proud flesh" (hypertrophic granulation tissue)
- ungual labial hypertrophy
- Nail base tender to palpation = bad ingrown
- Nail growth takes 9 months

TX:
- Chemical matrixectomy
  - Phenol (89%) & alcohol, or saline (P&A)
    - 3x 30 second applications of phenol
  - NaOH (10%) & acetic acid (5%) (vinegar)
    - less tissue breakdown compared to phenol

- o   Sterile technique not necessary
- o   Anesthetic block proximal to erythema to prevent failed block 2/2 to pH change
- Surgical:

Partial	Description
Frost	inverted "L" incision
Modified Frost	curved incision
Winograd	longitudinal wedge, excising nail matrix
Plastic lip	excision of pie shaped wedge of tissue from side of toe to treat hypertrophy of ungualabia

Total	Description
Zadik	avulse nail plate, two incisions from the corners of eponychium extending proximally. Distal strip of eponychium trimmed.
Kaplin	same as Zadik except excise entire matrix down to periosteum
Suppan	avulse nail, matrix is excised under the eponychium WITHOUT any incisions

Onychomycosis, tines unguium, dermatophyte of nail

- Most common infection of nail

ET:
- Offending agent (trauma) can cause keratin to build up under nail, which is breeding ground for fungus to grow
- Offending dermatophytes (fungus):
  - o   T rubrum (60%)
  - o   T mentagrophytes (20%)
  - o   E floccosum

RF:
- 30-60% originates from tinea pedis from surrounding skin
- Repeated nail trauma
- Environmental factors:
  - o   Occlusive footwear
  - o   Swimmer
  - o   Locker room exposure (shared shower areas)
  - o   Humidity
- Medical conditions:
  - o   DM
  - o   Immunosuppression (HIV)
  - o   positive family history
  - o   Vascular disease
  - o   Obesity

EP:
- 2-8%, older age group
- 25-30% of cases thought to be onychomycosis contain no active infection (PAS and culture negative
- an additional 30-40% of cases show onychomycosis but only as secondary phenomenon

NH:
- Can be a reservoir for dermatomycoses (tinea pedis) and spread to the skin
- Limit mobility —> venous stasis and diabetic foot ulcers
- Risk —> dystrophic nails —> ingrown toenail —> infection

CP:

Type*	Fungus	Details

Type*	Fungus	Details
Distal lateral subungual onychomycosis (DLSO)	T. rubrum	Most common DISTAL and lateral nail involvement without proximal nail involvement
Superficial white onychomycosis (SWO)	T. mentagrophytes	10%
Proximal subungual onychomycosis (PSO)	T. rubrum	least common immunocompromised begins in lunula and matrix
Endonyx onychomycosis (EO)	T. soudanense	involves nail plate WITHOUT hyperkeratosis and concurrent infection of nail bed
Candidal onychomycosis		

*Any can progress to total dystrophic onychomycosis
DX:

	Technique	Other
Culture (DTM-dermatophyte test medium)	Grow and ID living organisms from tissue sample	Poor sensitivity, high false negatives. Takes 4 weeks to issue final report
KOH (potassium hydroxide)	Clean nail with 70% ethyl alcohol, obtain as close to cuticle as possible Can add DMSO	poor sensitivity, tech dependent Does not identify species of fungus Better for tinea infections involving skin.
PAS (periodic acid Schiff)	Can combine with GMS stain for better sensitivity & specificity. Tissue is processed as a traditional biopsy, special stains are performed, and the sample is reviewed by a pathologist	Much more rapid than culture and KOH (takes only 24-48 hrs) Identifies actual species of fungus **Most sensitive & specific test**, provides additional information other than just offending agent
Mass spectrometry	"weigh" molecules in organism after blasting with laser	NOT good for fungi. Good only for yeast and bacterial infection
Molecular diagnostics	Identify organisms via DNA or RNA, as genetics are unaffected by environment. Identify via "high resultion melt technology" to measure the temperature at which the DNA breaks down	Results in 2-3 days NOT useful for bacteria, as too many probes are needed. Good for onychomycosis using 3 probes: dermatophyte, candida, saprophyte. The "future" of microbiological diagnostics

TX:
Topical agents + systemic therapy yield best results
- *Terbinafine + amorolfine 5% lacquer*

Resolution when 1) lack clinical sign 2) negative culture or microscopy results
- Nail avulsion-manual with nail nippers or chemical
- Oral therapy-risk hepatotoxicity, drug-drug interactions, risk relapse
- Topical treatment
  - Indicated for mild cases <50% involvement when only a few digits are affected
  - Difficult to penetrate nail
  - Lacquer leaves a water insoluble film that continuously releases medication into nail plate
  - More effective after initial debridement of nail
- Photodynamic therapy (after removing nail and hyperkeratotic material), Diode laser
- Home remedies: tea tree oil, Vicks vapor rub (camphor), apple cider vinegar

PO Antifungals

Drug name	SE	MOA	Dosage	Misc

Terbinafine HCl Lamisil ®	Hepatotoxic, (must order LFT/CBC) **Metallic taste**	inhibits squalene epoxidase (inhibits fungal cell wall formation)	250mg QD x 12 weeks (90 days)	Most potent against dermatophyte -Superior to itraconazole for tx of onychomycosis -least SE
Itraconazole Sporanox ®	Hepatotoxic, cP450 —> caution with oral contraceptives		200mg QD x 12 weeks (3 months), pulse dosing*	Dermatophytes and nondermatophyte, pregnancy category C
Fluconazole Diflucan ®	Renal		200mg QD	
Griseofulvin Grifulvin V ®	renal, hepatic	binds to microtubule to inhibit mitosis		

*pulse dosing: 3 x (200mg PO BID x1 week, 3 weeks off)

Topical antifungals

Drug name	Trade name	Dosage	Misc
Efinconazole	Jublia ®		Topical 10% solution FDA approved for onychomycosis
Clotrimazole solution		10mg TOP QD	Solution for nail
Ketoconazole		200mg TOP BID	
Ciclopirox	Penlac ®		8% lacquer, first FDA approved for onychomycosis 5.5-8.5% cure rate
Clotrimazole cream		1% cream	Cream for tinea pedis
Econazole	Spectazole®	1% cream	Cream for tinea pedis
Efinaconazole			Triazole antifungal
Amorolfine	Loceryl		Best cure rates in phase III clinical trials
Tavaborole	Kerydin ®		Boron-containing compound (5% oxaborole) leads to greater ability to penetrate keratin Broad spectrum against dermatophytes, yeast, mold FDA approved July 2014
Nyastatin and triamcinolone	Mycalog		tx for candidiasis: nyastatin kills the fungus, triamcinolone relieves the inflammation

IV antifungal

Drug name	SE	MOA	Dosage	Misc
Amphotericin B		antibiotic antifungal	QD	For severe fungal infections

Psoriasis
CP: PROXIMAL nail involvement, well defined patches of erythema (eczema is ill defined)

Onychodystrophy
- A condition of nails 2/2 to a disease
- Brittle nails where the keratin layers are separated

Onychauxis
- Thickened nail

Subungual hematoma
DX:
- XR to r/u digital fracture
- Biopsy to r/o malignant melanoma
TX:
- <25% = trephination using 18 gauge needle or #11 blade
  - >25% or nail fold involved = avulse nail, explore nail bed, suture close
- Open fracture
  - Lavage
  - debridement of bony fragments
  - Rx antibiotics

Bone Disease & Bone/Soft Tissue Tumors

RANK/RANKL (increase osteoclast) & OPG (decrease osteoclast) system influenced by:
- CNS—leptin decreases bone formation
- Endocrine-estrogen increases OPG
- PTH-decreases OPG
- Mechanical stress-increases OPG, increases bone formation
- NO low dose = anabolic, high dose = bone resorption

Stages of Bone healing
- Clinical healing: healing of pain and swelling
- Radiographic healing: healing of 3 of 4 cortices
- Wolff's law: bone will adapt to a load/pressure

Stage	Duration	Processes	Timing
1) Inflammatory	10%	-Pain, hyperemia, edema, -Differentiation of MSC into osteoblast & chondrocyte -Induction of growth factors	hours-1 week
Induction		Inflammation/edema	24 hours
Hematoma		Fibroblast, platelet differentiation	
2) Reparative/regenerative	40%	-Hematoma becomes invaded by fibroblasts —> bone callus -Capillary budding	
Soft callus		Cartilage	2-4 weeks
Hard callus		Calcification	6-8 weeks
3) Remodeling	70%	Osteoclast/osteoblast + Wolff's law	6 weeks-years

Two types of bone healing

- **3 Components of bone healing:** 1) vasculature 2) stability 3) nutrition
- **ORIF:** Requires 1) immobilization and 2) compression

	Primary/membranous/direct healing	Secondary/spontaneous/indirect/enchondral healing
Formation of bone	1) **Contact healing** (Haversian remodeling): when <0.1mm between fragments. Cutting cone- tip of osteoclasts in front, osteoblasts in back laying down concentric lamellar bone—> direct formation of new bone 2) **Gap healing**: bone deposition 90 deg to orientation of bone fragments, woven bone	Formation of **BONE CALLUS** (cartilaginous/fibrous tissue) resorption of callus —> wide gap filling of gap with cortical bone via Haversian remodeling
Callus formation	None	Callus formation
Fracture site	Good opposition, rigid fixation	Motion
Healing	More desirable method	Less desirable method

Types of bone

Woven	Lamellar
unorganized collagen fibers	parallel alignment
mechanically weak	mechanically strong
produced when osteoid produced rapidly	replaces woven bone

Zones of epiphyseal growth plate

Zone	Description	Location on epiphysis
Zone of proliferation/growth	chrondrocyte replication	closest to head (epiphysis)
Zone of maturation	chrondrocyte hypertrophy (enlargement), weak due to loss of intracellular matrix	
Zone of transformation	chondrocytes become calcified	
Zone of provisional calcification	between growth plate and metaphysis	closest to shaft

Nonunion

ET:

- **Comorbidities:** DIABETES, osteoporosis, hyperPTH, vitamin D deficiency, osteogenesis imperfecta, PVD, osteomyelitis
- **Social:** smoking, poor nutritional status (gastric bypass), poor bone quality, infection, ETOH consumption, history of excessive immobilization
- **Medications**: chronic steroid use (methotrexate), NSAIDs, immunosuppressants, chemotherapy,
- **Surgical:** poor joint prep, poor fixation, premature weight bearing or activity, prolonged NWB, hardware explant

DX:
Bone scan will show increased uptake for hypertrophic nonunion
- Indium 111 scan to r/o OM (will be negative if nonunion)
- Metabolic bone profile:
    - Vit D, Ca2+, thyroid panel (PTH, T3/T4)
    - if PTH low, not enough osteoclastic activity

TX:
Conservative:
- Oral calcitonin (inhibit osteoclast activity)
- Functional bracing
- **Bone stimulator**
    - <u>Mechanism</u>: electroNEGATIVE charge (5-20 microamperes) to stimulate bone growth at areas of growth and repair
    - <u>Duration</u>: 3-6 months
    - <u>Contraindication</u>: not for use in synovial pseudoarthrosis, gaps >1cm or >50% of bone diameter
    - invasive, semi-invasive, noninvasive
    - pulsed electromagnetic fields (PEMF), capacitive coupling (CC), combined magnetic field (CMF), low-intensity pulsed ultrasound (LIPUS)
- PRP
    - extracorporeal shockwave therapy (ESWT)

Surgical:
- **Grafts**
    - Bone graft-small defect
    - Intercalary graft-fresh frozen femoral head, <5cm
    - Trabecular cage
    - Vascularized graft-large defects 10-40cm, fibular free graft

Cancellous vs cortical graft healing

	Re-vasc	Growth pattern	Remodeling	Ostecytes	Strength
Cancellous	2 weeks	GAIN strength	completely	more	inferior
Cortical	2 months	LOOSE strength first 6 mo, progressively weaker	incompletely with necrotic pockets	less	superior structural strength

Stages of bone graft healing

	Stage	Activity	Osteobiologic
1	Vascular ingrowth	1-2 weeks	
2	Osteogenesis	**Osteoblasts** from the bone graft cause bone growth	
3	Osteoinduction	Regular bone growth MANY growth factors	**BMP** stimulates osteoblast production (FDA approved) **MSC allograft** **PRP**-provides growth factors **BMA**-provides MSC
4	Osteoconduction	Bone graft serves as "**scaffold/framework**" for osteoblasts to "conduct" and spread	**ceramic/bioactive glass**-osteoconductive, osteoinductive, antibacterial **DBM**-some osteoindcution
5	Graft remodeling	Via Wolff's law	

Osteobiologics summary

51

	Details
PRP	buffy coat (leukocyte rich)
	plasma based (leukocyte poor), better for OA treatment
	many methods of delivery-activated vs non-activated, platelet concentration
Stem cell	autologous
	allogenic
Cartiform	chondral mesh of Osteochondral allograft
Biocartilage	ECM scaffold for cells to augment microfractured defect
Arthroflex	Soft tissue scaffold

- **Ex Fix**
  - Decreased soft tissue dissection
  - Can be used with infection
  - Pain at pin site: infection OR loosening
  - Dynamization: before ex fix removal, pins are loosened and patient allowed to WB
    - ▢ Axial load without distraction strengthens bone, induces callus formation, faster healing time
  - Piezogenic effect: stress generates electric potentials in bone results in callus formation
- **Calandruccio triangular compression device**
  - Tri-planar compression
  - External frame good for ankle arthrodesis
  - one pin through tibia, one through talus

Weber and Cech classification for Nonunions (Pseudoarthroses)

Nonunion type	Freq	Description	Cause	Treatment
Hypertrophic/hyp ervascular	90%	**elephant foot**-LARGE callus, best chance healing **horse foot**-POOR callus **oligotrophic**-NO callus	adequate biology	good chance of healing. stable fixation via splint/ORIF
Atrophic/ Avascular/nonreac tive	10%	**atrophic**-fragment ends become atrophic **comminuted**-necrotic intermediate fragment **defect**-loss of fragments two ends are too far apart **torsion wedge**-intermediate fragment healed only to one of the main fragments	poor biology, impaired nutrients.	debridement, decortication, bone graft + mechanical stability

Complication	Characteristic	Treatment
Delayed union	No evidence of union for 6-9 months	immobilization
Nonunion	No evidence of union for >9 months (90 days for Medicare)	bone stim, bone graft
Malunion	When bone is reduced and heals in an improper position	
Pseudo-arthrosis	Fibrocartilaginous surface at bone fracture site, joint space contains synovial fluid	operation

Osteonecrosis
- Ischemic death of bone and bone marrow

ET:
- Trauma, alcoholism
- Methylmethacrylate (from hip implants)

CP:
- Osteoarthritis
- Freiberg's disease (epiphyseal osteonecrosis)
- Bone infarct
    - o Serpiginous calcification (diametaphyseal osteonecrosis)
    - o Asymptomatic
    - o Know the image!

DX:
- Bone scintigraphy, MRI, CT

Osteochondrosis
- disease of growth center-epiphysis or apophysis
-
    - Degeneration/necrosis followed by regeneration/recalcification
    - not to be confused with osteochondral defect (OCD) of talus

CP:
- LEADS TO OSTEONECROSIS
    - True osteonecrosis: Freiberg's, Mueller-Weiss, Kohler's
- XR: Fragmentation and sclerosis
- **Windswept deformity**
    - o Physeal osteochondrosis
    - o One knee valgus, other knee varus
    - o Treat with serial casting

Osteochondrosis/osteonecrosis

	Bone affected	Description
Kohler's disease	Navicular	Osteochondrosis, "coin sign", "coin on edge" or "silver dollar sign"-wafer thin flattened navicular bone mostly in boys 3-6 y.o., self limiting, TX: orthoses, NSAIDs
Freiberg's infraction	2nd MT	Osteochondrosis of 2nd MT head
Mueller-Weiss	navicular	adult osteochondrosis of navicular
Buschke disease	cuneiform	Osteonecrosis
Sever's apophysitis/Sever's disease	Calcaneus (osteochondrosis)	ET: Repetitive stress, overuse with damage and inflammation of the calcaneal apophysis (traction of Achilles), equinus Soccer or basketball player Shoegear irritation DX: pain with **SQUEEZE** (lateral compression) EP: 8-12 years old NH: resolves when the apophysis fuses with the body of the calcaneus (14-16 y.o.)
Iselin's disease	5th MT base	Apophysitis (osteochondrosis) of the base of the 5th MT
Osgood Schlatter	Tibial tubercle	Osteochondrosis, due to excessive traciton of patellar ligament Boys 11-15 y.o., basketball
Blount's disease	Medial tibial plafond	Osteochondrosis leading to bowlegged, African American predilection

Legg Calve Perthes disease	femoral head	Ostechondrosis 3-12 MOST COMMON OSTEOCHONDROSIS
Diaz/Mouchet	Talus	
Thiemann's	phalanges	
Lewin	distal tibia	
Ritter	proximal fibular head	
Treve	fibular sesamoid	
Renandier	tibial sesamoid	
Lance	cuboid	
Assmann	1st MT head	

Freiberg's infraction, AVN of 2nd MT head, osteochondrosis of metatarsal head

ET:
- Fracture of 2nd MT head
- An osteochondrosis/osteonecrosis (damage to growth center, vascular supply of bone) of 2nd MT head due to acute injury or repetitive micro trauma at an open physis.
- Trauma —> vascular injury —> AVN —> joint degeneration

EP: Adolescence to 20's (peak 12-14 y.o.)

NH: joint degeneration —> chronic OA-like pain

RF: repetitive microtrauma, vascular, long/PF'ed 2nd MT/short 1st MT, shoegear

CP: "Young female athlete with MT pain"

Radiograph:
- Flattened MT head
- "joint space widening and subchondral sclerosis"

Smillie classification:

	Description	Treatment
0	Normal radiograph	—
1	**Epiphysis fissure fracture**, joint space widening	immobilization
2	**Central depression** of MT head	
3	**Lateral projections**, *"Crescent sign"*	
4	Fracturing of the lateral projections, loose bodies	DFWO at base, shortening MT osteotomy, interpositional arthroplasty, resectional arthroplasty, arthrodesis, partial MT head resection, OATS
5	Flattened MT head	DFWO at base, shortening MT osteotomy, interpositional arthroplasty, resectional arthroplasty, arthrodesis, partial MT head resection, OATS

TX:

Conservative:
- Immobilization with below knee cast/removable cast boot
- Orthotic with MT bar
- Wide toe box, rigid shank, rocker bottom

Surgical:
- Distal MT osteotomy, implant arthroplasty, MT head remodeling, resection arthroplasty
- **Interpositional grafting**-insert cancellous bone graft to restore contour of MT head
- **Rotational osteotomy**-excise damaged cartilage and rotate plantar MT head dorsally to allow cartilage to articulate with proximal phalanx
- OATS-donor site @ TNJ, under spring ligament (good curve)

BONE TUMORS
- Primary or metastatic

DX: biopsy

CP:
- Lytic bone lesions: FOGMACHINES
- Sclerotic bone lesions: VINDICATE

Patterns of destruction

Type	Description	Severity of aggression
Geographic	well defined with short zone of transition from normal to abnormal bone.	slow growing
Moth-eaten	longer zone of transition	more aggressive
Permeative	poorly defined lesion margins	most aggressive

Periosteal reactions

Severity	Type	Description
Least severe	Buttressing	thick periostitis, slow growing tumor presses against periosteum, thickening of cortex
	Lamellated/onion skin	multiple layers of new periosteal bone
	Sunburst	delicate rays
	Hair-on-end/spiculated	similar to sunburst but rays are parallel and perpendicular to underlying bone
Most severe	Codman's triangle/Codman's angle	triangle elevation of periosteum with buttress

Bone tumors (malignant)
Osteosarcoma
- *Most common malignant* bone tumor
- EP: 20-30 y.o. or teenagers during growth spurt
  - CP:
    - Codman's triangle/Codman's angle

Osteochondroma vs. subungual exostosis

	Osteochondroma	Subungual exostosis
Etiology	Disruption in development of cortex	Trauma
Progression	Slower growing	Slow pre-puberty, rapid in adolescence
Age	Adolescent	20-40 yo
Radiograph	Cancellous bone	Cortex confluent with underlying bone
Histology	Hyaline cartilage cap	Fibrocartilage cap
Size	Can be much larger than exostosis	

Bone tumors (benign)

Tumor	Details
Osteochondroma	• **Most common** benign bone tumor • CP: Commonly subungual (confused with subungual exostosis) —> pincer nail • Mushroom/mound-bony outgrowth with cartilaginous cap (most common), looks like heterotopic ossification • Pedunculated-with a stalk • Sessile-broad based • **Osteochondromatosis**-multiple osteochondromas
Osteoma	Located in skull, periosteum XR: osteochondroma with cartilaginous cap
Enostosis	Bone island
Osteoblastoma	AKA giant osteoid osteoma, night pain NOT relieved by aspirin
Osteoid osteoma	*Night pain relieved by aspirin* Dense sclerotic bone surrounding a lytic, lucent central nidus
Enchondroma	Predilection for phalanges Tumor of hyaline cartilage Many areas of decreased density, flecked appearance **Ollier's disease (enchondromatosis)**-multiple enchondromas **Maffuci's syndrome**-enchondromas associated with soft tissue hemangioma and telangiectasias
Unicameral bone cyst (UBC)	"FALLEN FRAGMENT SIGN" In calcaneus Thin sclerotic margin
Aneurysmal bone cyst (ABC)	filled with blood
Giant Cell tumor	similar to ABC
Intra-osseus lipoma	Calcaneal bone cyst with intra-osseus calcification
Fibrous dysplasia	Ground glass, more centered
Ossifying fibroma	Predilection for mandible
Non-ossifying fibroma/fibrocortical defect	Connective tissue: muscle/tendon insertion. Painless, in children
Fibro osseus defect	incidental finding, off-centered tumor in tibia in child
Bone infarct	Tibial tumor centered in skeletally mature
Brown tumor	AKA hyperparathyroidism, osteoclastoma
Paget's disease	• Associated with osteosarcoma, chondrosarcoma, fibrosarcoma • Stages: 1) osteoclastic, 2) mixed osteoclast/osteoblast activity, 3) osteoblastic, 4) malignant degeneration

Bone Disease Summary[52]

Bone disease
Melorheostosis -wax flowing down candle -wavy inner or outer cortex

[52] Images taken from Christman, Robert. Foot and ankle radiology. Lippincott Williams & Wilkins, 2014.

Ricket's, osteomalacia
-vitamin D deficiency
-bowing, looser zone, milkman zone, metaphyseal cupping/fraying
-**White line of Frankel**-transverse line of increased density
-**Scurvy line**-dark line
Scurvy
-2/2 vitamin C deficiency
-**Wimburger's sign**-ring epiphysis
-**Pelken's spur**-beaky outgrowth in scurvy
Osteopetrosis, "marble bone disease"
-bone wtithin bone appearance
Osteopoikilosis
-multiple bone islands

SOFT TISSUE TUMORS

DX:
- Biopsy
  - Incisional biopsy-cutting and removing part of the lesion
  - Excision biopsy-remove the entire lesion
- Physical exam:
  - Motile = benign, superficial
  - Trans-illumination

TX:
Excisional biopsy
- Length to width ratio: 3:1

Soft tissue tumors (benign) (87%)

Degenerative origin:	
Ganglion cyst AKA mucinous cyst (on the toes/nail fold)	Most common benign soft tissue tumor in FOOT (lipoma MC soft tissue tumor in BODY)
	ET:
	-Union of small cysts due to DEGENERATION of soft tissue
	-Repetitive microtrauma (could be 2/2 to bony exostosis), mucosal degeneration
	CP: Occur at joint or tendon sheath
	Baker's cyst-at popliteal fossa
	DX: transillumination—entire mass will light up
	TX: aspiration, excision with drain (prevent hematoma formation, prevent infection)
Plantar fibroma/plantar fibromatosis AKA Lederhaus disease	CP:
	-Usually at proximal/central plantar aponeurosis
	-Non-mobile, not soft/squishy
	-Associated with: **Dupuytren** contracture (flexion contracture of hand), **Peyronies** disease (curved penis, nodules on penis)
	TX: Offload, steroid injection, excision (high recurrence)
Synovial origin:	
Pigmented villonodular synovitis (PVNS)	Intra-articular tumor of single joint
	MC soft tissue tumor to metastasize to bone
Giant cell tumor of tendon sheath (GCTTS)	Extra-articular tumor of tendon sheath

Synovial sarcoma	MC malignancy in foot
Other origin:	
Leiomyoma	Angioleiomyoma Pilar leiomyoma-arrector pilli
Neurilemoma	Nerve sheath tumors
Schwannoma	Arise from Schwann cell of nerve sheath
Neurofibroma	Arise from superficial cutaneous nerves
Glomus tumor	Most commonly found in nail bed Pain on palpation
Lipoma	Mostly on dorsum of foot Transillumination
Xanthoma	Cholesterol rich deposits (Achilles T)
Hemangioma	Calcification of vv

Soft tissue tumors (Malignant)

Type	Description
Synovial sarcoma	Deep, painless
malignant lymphoma	usually known history of lymphoid disease
Fibrosarcoma	

Limb length discrepancy (LLD)
ET:
- Structural-unequal bone length
- Functional-contracture in lower limb joint. Rigid or dynamic (cerebral palsy, hemiplegia)

EP: 40%-70%

DX: ASIS to medial malleolus, line up medial malleoli

CP:
- Pronation/pes planus on long side, supination on short side
- Hip flexion on long side
- Pelvic tilt is MOST COMMON compensation for MINOR degrees of deformity
- Knee flexion is most common for SEVERE degrees of deformity

Compensations for limb length discrepancy

Compensation type	Direction of Compensation
Pelvic tilt	Toward short side
Anterior sacrum	Toward short side
Sacral rotation	Toward long side
Pelvic shift	Toward long side
Lumbar scoliosis	Convex spine to short side
Knee flexion	Long side

Compensation type	Direction of Compensation
Genu recurvatum	Short side
Subtalar pronation	Long side
Subtalar supination	Short side
Ankle plantarflexion	Short side

First Ray Pathology

Hallux abducto valgus (HAV) (bunion), hallux IPJ (HIPJ) abductus, hallux abductus interphalangeus, hallux valgus interphalangeus (HVI)

ET/RF:

POSITIONAL:
- Hypermobile 1st ray (normal is +/- 5mm) <--> increased IM angle --> overpronation —> unable to activate windlass mechanism --> unable to form a rigid level —>unlocked MTJ —> calcaneal eversion —>unstable PL
  - o Metatarsus primus varus —> shorter lever arm —> transverse migration of 1st MT (1st MT escape)
  - o Metatarsus primus elevatus (MPE)
  - o Reverse windlass mechanism-a lowered arch results in a plantarflexed hallux. Windlass unable to overcome ground reactive force on first ray. Foot is unable to resupinate.
- Biomechanical abnormality (tibia torsion, genu varum/valgum, MT adductus, pes planus, forefoot valgus)
  - o Equinus
    - ☐ Inverts 1st MT, reduced influence of PL (Johnson et al JFAS 2005[53])
    - ☐ Increased forefoot pressure —> opposes stability of peroneus longus —> foot overpronates to compensate for lack of DF —> hypermobile 1st ray
- Frontal plane deformity
  - o Eversion/pronation/valgus rotation of 1st MT
  - o medial eminence is dorsomedial aspect of 1st MTPJ

STRUCTURAL:
- 1st ray insufficiency—> imbalance of forces between 1st and 2nd MT
  - o Effects: hypermobile 1st ray, short 1st MT
  - o Symptoms: overpronation, callus sub 2nd, pain 2nd MT base, 2nd MT shaft thickening
- Atavistic cuneiform: medial deviation of medial cuneiform causing an adducted 1st MT
  - o Controversial
  - o Argued to be the source of metatarsus primus varus deformity
  - o Can be deceptively present due to position of first ray (MPE, pronation/supination)[54]
  - o Medial cuneiform articulation with 1st MT can be rounded or trapezoidal (worse for surgery, shortens 1st ray)
  - o Can skew 1st ray radiographic measurements[55]
  - o Various shapes of 1st TMT articulation

  - o Cuneiform shape: oblique, curved, 2nd MT base facet, reverse slope

- 1st MT head shape[56]:
  - o Round (greatest risk for HAV and recurrence) 2/2 to pronated, metatarsus primus varus/metatarsus primus elevatus deformity

---

[53] Johnson, Cherie H., and Jeffrey C. Christensen. "Biomechanics of the first ray part V: The effect of equinus deformity: A 3-dimensional kinematic study on a cadaver model." The Journal of foot and ankle surgery 44.2 (2005): 114-120.

[54] Sanicola, Shawn M., Thomas B. Arnold, and Lawrence Osher. "Is the radiographic appearance of the hallucal tarsometatarsal joint representative of its true anatomical structure?." Journal of the American Podiatric Medical Association 92.9 (2002): 491-498.

[55] Miller, SJ THE FIRST METATARSOCUNEIFORM JOINT: Analysis and Clinical Application, Podiatry Institute Update 1995

[56] Okuda, Ryuzo, et al. "The shape of the lateral edge of the first metatarsal head as a risk factor for recurrence of hallux valgus." The Journal of Bone & Joint Surgery 89.10 (2007): 2163-2172.

- o   Square (least risk), chevron (square with central ridge)
- o   **Lateral round sign**-roundness of lateral MT head 2/2 valgus rotation of 1st MT (Okuda et al, JBJS 2007[57])

OTHER:
- • Iutrogenic
  - o   Plantar fasciotomy leading to hypermobile 1st ray
  - o   FHL T transfer—> removes stabilizing force during mid stance
  - o   Tibial sesamoidectomy
  - o   PL —>PB tenodesis
- • Pathological: neuromuscular disorder, inflammatory arthropathy
- • Genetics
- • Inflammatory disease
- • Muscle imbalance at 1st MTPJ

EP:
- • 33% of adults
- • Females >> males

NH:
- • 1st MTPJ is a ginglymoarthroidal joint:
  - o   Ginglymo: **sagittal** motion first 20-30 DF
  - o   Arthroidal: **transitional gliding** motion 30-60 DF
- • 2 axes of 1st MTPJ:
  - o   1) Transverse (allows for sagittal motion)
  - o   2) Sagittal (allows for transverse motion)
- • More sagittal plane ROM at medial arch than ankle (Lundgren et al 2008[58])
- • Contribution to 1st ray sagittal ROM (Roling et al, JFAS 2002[59])
  - o   **NCJ-50%**
  - o   **FMCJ-41%**
  - o   **TN-9%**

HAV stages:

	Details	Root, Orien, Weed Stage
I	**Lateral shift of proximal phalanx:** (subclinical subluxation of 1st MTPJ)	1st ray hypermobility
II	**Hallux abducts:** intrinsics/extrinsics lose normal vector-FHB and FHL lateralize their kinematic vector	MTJ instability
III	**Medial buckling of 1st MT head (metatarsus primus varus):** inc IMA Hallux rotates in valgus position (tibial sesamoid position > 3)	calcaneal eversion
IV	**Subluxed/dislocated 1st MPJ**	PL instability

CP:
- • Painful bump
  - o   Adults-pain due to longstanding OA
  - o   Juvenile-pain due to medial bump rubbing on shoe
- • Hallux abductus interphalangeus deformity: abduction @ HIPJ, best tx: arthrodesis
- • Hallux overlapping 2nd digit 2/2 to hypermobile 1st ray
- • Pronated foot
- • Ankle equinus

---

[57] Okuda, Ryuzo, et al. "The shape of the lateral edge of the first metatarsal head as a risk factor for recurrence of hallux valgus." The Journal of Bone & Joint Surgery 89.10 (2007): 2163-2172.

[58] Lundgren, P., et al. "Invasive in vivo measurement of rear-, mid-and forefoot motion during walking." Gait & posture 28.1 (2008): 93-100.

[59] Roling, Brian A., Jeffrey C. Christensen, and Cherie H. Johnson. "Biomechanics of the first ray. Part IV: the effect of selected medial column arthrodeses. A three-dimensional kinematic analysis in a cadaver model." The Journal of foot and ankle surgery 41.5 (2002): 278-285

- Lesser digit contractures
- Lateral displacement of sesamoids
- Callus sub 2nd MT
- Hallux position: congruent vs. deviated vs. subluxed

DX:

Weight bearing:
- Hallux purchase (paper pulling test), EHL contracture
- Increased deformity indicates hypermobile 1st ray

NonWB:
- Root test-normal test by grabbing 1st/2nd MT head (with ankle/STJ neutral)
- Dynamic Hicks test-(with ankle/STJ neutral, DF hallux between 2nd and 3rd digit, 1st and 3rd hold on to first MT head while testing for hypermobility)
- Jack's test-AKA windlass mechanism
- 1st MTPJ ROM
- Squeeze test-check for reducibility of IM angle
  - Reducible = positional, not structural etiology
- Tracking vs trackbound
  - **Tracking**-deviation of hallux only towards end of DF/PF ROM
  - **Trackbound**-"C-shaped ROM"—deviation of hallux throughout entire ROM

XR:

Type of deformity	Angles
Structural	PASA + DASA > HAA
Positional	PASA + DASA < HAA
Combined	PASA + DASA >>> HAA

- Sesamoid position
  - Weakness of AP view: sesamoids appear to shift laterally into the inter metatarsal space with valgus rotation of 1st MT
    - in reality, sesamoid shift appears to drift due to valgus frontal ROTATION of 1st MT, not lateral displacement of sesamoids
    - sesamoids maintain same distance to 2nd MT 2/2 tethering effect of adducturo hallucis and deep transverse MT ligament
    - NO correlation with sesamoid position in sesamoid axial view
- Intraoperatively: check for hypermobility by:
  - Using live fluoroscopy
  - Selectively pinning joints

TX:
- Conservative:
  - Wider toe box, bunion pad, RICE, NSAIDs, steroid injection
  - Orthoses-good only for 6 months
- Surgery: Best treatment for long term pain relief (JAMA 2001[60])

Surgical goals
1) Correction of HAA: joint congruency of 1st MT head relative to proximal phalanx
   a. Relieves retrograde buckling generated by hallux which can cause "spontaneous", "unpredictable" changes in frontal plane correction of metatarsal
2) SESAMOID POSITION, when uncorrected, can be a risk factor for recurrence[61]
   a. If uncorrected, consider additional release of dorsolateral capsule of 1st MTPJ as well as release of lateral collateral ligament
   b. For Austin procedure, sesamoids iatrogenically sublux medial to the median crista 2/2 lateral release and medial capsular plication.
   c. Risks recurrence over time as sesamoids drift laterally 2/2 pull of FHB to return to their anatomic position in the sesamoidal grooves of a pronated metatarsal
3) Lateral release:
   a. Adductor tendon

[60] Torkki, Markus, et al. "Surgery vs orthosis vs watchful waiting for hallux valgus: a randomized controlled trial." Jama 285.19 (2001): 2474-2480.

[61] Okuda, Ryuzo, et al. "Postoperative incomplete reduction of the sesamoids as a risk factor for recurrence of hallux valgus." The Journal of Bone & Joint Surgery 91.7 (2009): 1637-1645.

    b. Lateral capsule
    c. Transverse MT ligament
    d. Lateral (fibular) sesamoid ligament
    e. FHB tendon
    f. Fibular sesamoidectomy
4) Procedure selection
    a. <u>Positional deformity</u>: distal osteotomy
    b. <u>Structural deformity</u>: (large IM angle, rigid): proximal osteotomy/arthrodesis
    c. <u>Triplanar deformity</u>: correct all 3 planes
    d. Pick procedure, amount of lateral release, based on severity of deformity
    e. "Difficult HAV" (other overlapping pathology): pes planus, hypermobility, MT adductus, DMAA (PASA), equinus.
        i. **All these factors are associated with juvenile HAV
5) Frontal plane correction[62]
    a. Medial translation of sesamoid s/p lateral release to give the "appearance" of a re-aligned sesamoid position doesn't correct a valgus rotated 1st MT
    b. FHB will eventually pull sesamoids back into 1st interspace, under the cristae
6) Complications (4-11%, up to 50% of all cases)
    a. Recurrence
    b. Revision surgery have poorer prognosis compared to primary repair
        i. Importance to RESTORE LENGTH of 1st MT

Algorithm for treatment of HAV based on staging (JFAS 2003[63])

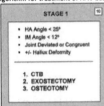
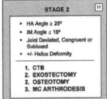
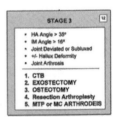

Summary of HAV Surgical Procedures[64]

	Indication	Procedure	Other
Capsule tendon balance (CTB) procedures:			
Silver		Bumpectomy, lateral release, medial capsular imbrication	Return to ambulation: as tolerated by pain
McBride		Silver + fibular sesamoidectomy + adductor hallucis tendon transfer (re-attached to medial capsule), capsulorraphy	

[62] Dayton, Paul, Merrell Kauwe, and Mindi Feilmeier. "Is Our Current Paradigm for Evaluation and Management of the Bunion Deformity Flawed? A Discussion of Procedure Philosophy Relative to Anatomy." The Journal of Foot and Ankle Surgery 54.1 (2015): 102-111.
[63] Vanore et al, Diagnosis and Treatment of First Metatarsophalangeal Joint Disorders. Section 1: Hallux Valgus, Journal of Foot and Ankle Surgery 2003, 42; 3:112-23
[64] Ryan, Jay D., Eugene D. Timpano, and Thomas A. Brosky. "Average Depth of Tarsometatarsal Joint for Trephine Arthrodesis." The Journal of Foot and Ankle Surgery 51.2 (2012): 168-171.

Modified McBride		No fibular sesamoidectomy to prevent hallux varus	
Hallux procedure			
Akin	Adducts hallux **Proximal**-DASA **Distal**-HIA	Closing lateral wedge resection of proximal phalanx (opening medial, apex lateral) + Silver	Cosmetic adjunct, Complication: transverse plane deformity
Keller	IMA > 15	Joint destructive: remove 1/3 base of prox phalanx + lat release. -corrects IM angle which treats the hypermobility of 1st ray -Add hemi implant to prevent shortening tx hallux rigidus -tx chronic hallux ulcer	-For elderly/less active. -Risks: hallux instability, cock up hallux (FHL transection), **short toe**, contracture, lose push-off strength, lose hallux purchase, **transfer metatarsalgia**, impaired Windlass, transfer lesions sub 2nd MT
Head procedures, distal metatarsal osteotomy (DMO)		IMA CORRECTION—>WINDLASS ACTIVATED—>STABLE FIRST RAY	SE: MT head AVN, interdigital neuritis, joint stiffness 2/2 scarring from lateral release
Austin/chevron		-Chevron osteotomy -Lateral translation of capital fragment up to 50% -1mm lateral shift = 1 deg IMA correction	-no change in postop plantar pressures (still sub 2nd MT head) -limiting factor for correction: width of MT head -good for bump pain -**contraindication:** MTPJ pain
Youngswick	Shortens and plantarflexes	Chevron with removal of bone in dorsal arm	For MPE
Reverdin	PASA	Closing lateral wedge resection of MT head (lateral cortex intact) + Silver	
Reverdin Green	PASA	Closing lateral wedge preserving sesamoid apparatus	sesamoid preserved
Reverdin-Laird	PASA + IM	Reverdin-Green osteotomy through lateral cortex	sesamoid preserved
Reverdin-Todd	PASA + IM + plantarflexes	Reverdin-Laird osteotomy through plantar cortex	loss sesamoid
Watermann	Hallux limitus/rigidus	Removal of dorsal wedge plantar cortex intact	

Waternmann Green	Hallux limitus/rigidus	Watermann with preservation of sesamoid	
Neck procedures			
Peabody		Reverdin proximal to sesamoids	
Mitchell	IMA, MPE	removes medial shelf, shorten, PF MT head	
Hohmann	IMA, PASA, MPE	Reverdin with capital fragment PF & lateral shift	
Wilson	long 1st MT	SHORTENS with lateral displacement of head	
DRATO	IMA, PASA, PF 1st MT, hallux limitus	Derotational abductory transpositional osteotomy VERY UNSTABLE!!!	
Shaft procedures			
Scarf osteotomy	IMA	60 degree sideways "Z"	-Risk for *troughing* -following plantar slope will PF MT head -2 buried head screws
Mau/Ludloff	IMA	Mau: prox plantar—> distal dorsal Ludloff: prox dorsal—> distal plantar	
Kalish		Long dorsal arm Austin, 55 deg	able to insert 2 screws
Lambrinudi	MPE	Oblique cut at shaft	
Vogler		Offset V osteotomy with apex at metaphyseal diaphyseal junction. 40 degree cut	
Base procedures			

		MOA:	
Lapidus (first described by Albrecht, Kleinberg and Truslow) **Modified Lapidus:** 1st TMT fusion **True Lapidus:** fusion of 1st and 2nd TMT due to transverse hypermobility	IMA > 15 Hypermobile first ray, unstable medial column @ FMTCJ, MT adductus	**MOA:** -TRI-PLANAR correction -can increase medial arch height -met primus varus must be corrected to obtain satisfactory correction **Technique:** -Fusion of FMTCJ via currettage, but maintain subchondral plate. -Modified: lateral (linear) capsulotomy, medial (elliptical) capsulotomy -importance of FRONTAL plane correction -impingement of dorsolateral tuberosity of 1st MT base—>can shave off **Cons:** NWB for 6 weeks, nonunion, malunion (5.3%), **1st MT shortening**, NC joint arthritis, arthritis of lesser MCJ **Causes of nonunion** -smoking, poor nutritional status, poor bone quality -poor joint prep/poor fixation, poor postop care, prolonged NWB	-For moderate to severe deformity, recurrent HAV. -Can be used for flatfoot correciton Helps engage PL to stabilize med column (Christensen) Triplanar correction **Increases forefoot load sharing:** -decreases pressure sub 2nd MT head, and shifts pressure laterally to sub 5th -cross screws BEFORE plate - depth of 1st TMT joint: 3.2cm, 2nd: 2.7, 3rd: 2.4 (JFAS 2012 Ryan et al)
OBWO Crescentic (Trethowan)	lengthen MT	may DF or PF the MT, does not shorten MT NWB for 6-8 weeks	
CBWO **Oblique** (Juvara) 2) **Straight** (Loison Balacescu)	large IMA > 15 1 mm wedge = 3 deg correction in IMA	-types A, B, C -osteotomy perpendicular to MT shaft: DF of first ray -osteotomy perpendicular to WB surface: no change in sagittal plane **Risks:** #1: MPE! Unstable, NWB 2-3 wks, hinge break, shortening the MT, DF/PF MT	Axis guide: **Saggital:** perpendicular to WB surface -perpendicular to MT shaft will elevate -pependicular in opposite will PF (aim distally) **Frontal:** perpendicular to WB surface -axis point medially = PF axis point laterally = DF
Proximal Austin		shortens MT	
Logroscino	IMA, PASA	Reverdin + Loison Balacescu (opening ABductory wedge at base)	
Capsulotomies			
Washington monument		**TIGHTENS** medial capsulotomy, good frontal + transverse correction	
Lenticular		frontal + transverse correction removal of redundant medial capsule	
Inverted L		transverse correction removal of redundant medial capsule	
Mediovertical		resect redundant plantar capsule	

Blood supply to sesamoids:
- Proximal/distal medial branches coming off the 1st plantar MTA.

Hallux limitus/rigidus, aka metatarsus primus elevatus (MPE), aka dorsal bunion, hallux extensus
<65 degrees hallux DF

Hallux limitus/rigidus:
> *"Painful, acquired, arthritic condition of the 1st MTPJ, decreased sagittal plane motion"*

Metatarsus primus elevatus (MPE):
- DF 1st ray —> hallux tries to DF against elevated MT head —> arthritis of 1st MTPJ
- Fixed structural deformity OR functional positional state
- Controversial:
  a. No correlation, MPE corrected with dorsiflexion stress test (Coughlin et al, JBJS 2003[65])
  b. MPE >5mm could be considered predictive factor[66]
  c. Skewed measurements of MPE based on technique of taking lateral radiograph[67]

ET/RF:
1) STRUCTURAL-occuring during WB & NWB
   a. LONG 1st MT (overloaded 1st MTPJ, functions as DF 1st ray), Short 1st MT (FHB contracture)
   b. Metatarsus primus elevatus (MPE)
   c. Scarred joint capsule
   d. Contracted medial plantar fascia
   e. Hypertrophic sesamoids
   f. Weak peroneus longus
2) FUNCTIONAL-occuring WB when foot is loaded
   a. Overpronation/pes planus deformity/metatarsus primus elevatus (MPE)
   b. Hypermobile 1st ray
   d. Greater DF of 1st ray (hypermobility) results in less 1st MTPJ DF (Roukis et al, JAPMA 2005[68])
      i. DF 1st ray and PF proximal phalanx ==> DECREASED hallux DF
   e. Unlocked MTJ
   f. Early engagement of windlass mechanism
   g. FHL creates "jamming effect" (retrograde buckling of dorsal rim of proximal phalanx)
   h. FHB contracture + immobility of sesamoid apparatus
      i. inability for 1st MT to glide over sesamoid apparatus during propulsion
3) POST-TRAUMATIC
   a. Arthritis
   b. OCD
   c. 1st MPJ injury/fracture/hyperextension/hyperflexion (turf toe) leading to osteochondrosis
4) Metabolic
   a. OA/RA/gout
5) Neuromuscular
   a. FHB contracture + sesamoid degeneration/immobility
   b. Extrinsic/intrinsic muscle imbalance
6) Iatrogenic:
   a. Abnormal 1st MT elevation
   b. Joint fibrosis

EP: Female, 2nd most common 1st MTPJ pathology 2/2 to HAV
NH:
Drago, Orloff and Jacobs (1-4), Regnauld (1-3)

Regnauld	Symptom	Radiographic findings	Treatment

[65] Coughlin, Michael J., and Paul S. Shurnas. "Hallux rigidus." The Journal of Bone & Joint Surgery 85.11 (2003): 2072-2088
[66] Bouaicha, Samy, et al. "Radiographic analysis of metatarsus primus elevatus and hallux rigidus." Foot & ankle international 31.9 (2010): 807-814
[67] Christman, Robert A., et al. "Radiographic analysis of metatarsus primus elevatus: a preliminary study." Journal of the American Podiatric Medical Association 91.6 (2001): 294-299. APA
[68] Roukis, Thomas S. "Metatarsus primus elevatus in hallux rigidus: fact or fiction?." Journal of the American Podiatric Medical Association 95.3 (2005): 221-228

Stage 1: Functional limitus	Pain on END ROM Hallux equinus Hyperextension of IPJ Pronatory foot	NONE Metatarsus primus elevatus	Joint preserving
Stage 2: Joint adaptation	Limited ROM pain on end ROM Synovial membrane thickening	Joint space narrowing MT head flattening Small dorsal exostosis Subchondral eburnation-(sclerosis due to loss of cartilage)	Joint preserving
Stage 3: Arthrosis	Pain with ENTIRE ROM Crepitus	Dorsal osteophytes splint formation"	Joint preserving/destructive
Stage 4: Ankylosis	<10 degrees ROM Pain due to skin irritation or bursitis	Obliteration of joint space Excess osteophytosis	Joint destructive

Coughlin and Shurnas (0-4)[69]

Grade	Radiograph	Clinical	Dorsiflexion
0 "functional limitus"	normal	no pain, only dec ROM	as low as 40 deg
1	Osteophytes, no joint space narrowing		as low as 30 deg
2	<25% joint space narrowing		as low as 10 deg
3	>25% joint space narrowing	no pain mid-range	less than 10 deg
4	same as 3	pain mid-range	less than 10 deg

CP:
- <65 degrees hallux DF
  - NORMAL: 65-90 DF, >15 PF
  - 50-60 deg needed for gait
- Hallux extensus deformity-IPJ hyperextension due to inability of MT head to glide over sesamoid apparatus, 2/2 hyper mobility
  - Floating hallux
- *Hallux IPJ ulcer*
  - 1st MTPJ stiffness, pain aggravated by shoes
- Dorsal bony prominence (dorsal flag sign)
- Lateral foot pain 2/2 compensation
- Hallux equinus
  - Callus/pain sub 2nd MT, sub 4th MT 2/2 to compensatory forefoot inversion
- **Apropulsive gait**: overpronatory, forefoot inversion, early toe off, abductory/pronatory twist, shorter stride length, greater knee and hip flexion.

DX:

XR:
- MPE:
  - Seiberg index-comparison of dorsal cortex of 1st and 2nd MT in lateral view
  - Distance between metaphysis of MT neck NORMAL <8mm
  - 1st MT declination-normal 19-25 deg

[69] Coughlin, Michael J., and Paul S. Shurnas. "Hallux rigidus." The Journal of Bone & Joint Surgery 85.11 (2003): 2072-2088

- Subchondral sclerosis, joint space narrowing, osteophytosis, MT head flattening

TX:

Conservative:
- NSAIDs, wide toe-box shoe, rocker bottom shoe, stiff-soled shoe, corticosteroid injections (phosphate for joints), orthoses (only for functional hallux limitus) with Morton's extension

Surgery
- To relieve excessive joint compression
- Ensure mobility of plantar plate structures are adequate

Joint preserving:

Cheilectomy-take off 1/3 dorsal articular surface of MT head and prox phalanx
- o OK if joint space present
- o Can correct MPE by restoring 1st MTPJ ROM
- o **Grind test:** pressing on sesamoids while DF'ing hallux—if pain elicited, cheilectomy may not be effective
- o Effective when no MT deformity present, or else perform in conjunction with MT head procedure
- o Chondroplasty-fenestration (microfracture) of MT head to stimulate MSC to produce fibrocartilage (NOT HYALINE)

- Hyaluronate, NSAID s/p procedure:
  - o IMPROVES SYMPTOMS and DECREASE PAIN
    - ▢ Could be 2/2 to denervation
  - o Does NOT:
    - ▢ Address structural deformity
    - ▢ Prevent disease progression
    - ▢ Increase ROM

Joint Preserving Procedures

Indication: when patient has MPE

Risks:
- DO NOT perform in isolation!
- 1st MT shortening:
- Metatarsalgia 2/2 to altered MT parabola

Distal MT osteotomy aka 1st MT decompressional osteotomy	Description
Waterman	DFWO of MT neck
Waterman Green	preserves sesamoid apparatus, removes rectangular section of bone
Youngswick	remove bone in dorsal arm, also corrects for high IMA
Proximal plantar displacement osteotomy	corrects long MT
Reverdin	
Hohmann	

Phalangeal osteotomy	Description
Kessel and Bonney, Moberg	DFWO of proximal phalanx base Originally for adolescents Decompresses joint SE: sacrifices PF to gain DF
Regnauld (Mexican hat procedure)	peg in hole, loss of flexor function

Joint Destructive Procedures[70] [71]:

Joint destructive procedure	Details	
Keller	resect proximal phalanx	
Moberg	Osteotomy at base of proximal phalanx, with or without cheilectomy	
Heuter	complete resection of MT head also used to tx OM, pan MT head resection	
Valenti	Dorsal portions of proximal phalanx and 1st MT head removed	
Stone	-resect MT head -preserve sesamoids	
Mayo	-remove sesamoids	
Arthrodesis (McKeever)	GOLD STANDARD **Indication:** When <50% of articular cartilage remaining **Contraindicated:** MPE, long 1st MT **Pros:** 🗹 **Younger athletes:** maintains toe push off 🗹 **CORRECTS IMA w/o need for base osteotomy** (Cronin FAI 2006, JFAS 2014)	Fuse toe position: 1) Abducted/valgus 10 degrees 2) DF at 15 degrees (because 1st MT is declined at 15 degrees!!) NWB 4-6 wks SE: nonunion, mal-alignment, arthritis of hallux IPJ, hallux HT
Implant arthroplasty	**Hemi-**metallic Hemi-cap: minimal resection of bone (Kline 2014) **Total-**double stem flexible silicone hinge **Two-component**	**Purpose:** remove pain, NOT restore normal ROM **SE:** infection, implant failure, reactive synovitis/metallosis, silicone-induced synovitis -More prone to fail (compared to knee implants) due to small surface area of 1st MTPJ -Difficult to salvage due to bone loss
Interpositional arthroplasty	**Interposition of EHB and dorsal capsule sutured to plantar plate** Allograft, xenograft, or medial capsule into joint space Poor results	capsular imbrication purse-string/hour glass capsulorraphy U flap or V flap

Arthroplasty vs Arthrodesis

[70] Cronin, John J., et al. "Intermetatarsal angle after first metatarsophalangeal joint arthrodesis for hallux valgus." Foot & ankle international 27.2 (2006): 104-109
[71] Kline, Alex J., and Carl T. Hasselman. "Metatarsal head resurfacing for advanced hallux rigidus." Foot & ankle international (2013): 1071100713478930.

Arthroplasty	Arthrodesis
Better ROM, better flexibility	good for history of first ray instability
no need for postop NWB	postop NWB, risk nonunion, gait disturbance, IPJ arthritis
Weaker hallux propulsion	Better propulsion
1st MT shortening, hallux drift	no osteotomy needed at phalanx or 1st MT

JFAS Clinical Guideline Algorithm[72]

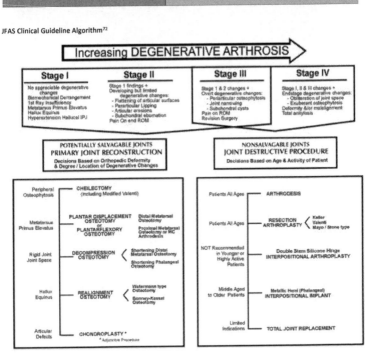

Hallux varus
ET/RF: Fibular sesamoidectomy, overtightening of capsule, over tightening bandage, staking the head, arthridities, congenital, neuromuscular, trauma, long 1st ray/hallux

CP: Medial deviation of great toe, IPJ bursitis, lesser toe adductus, hindfoot supination

Type 1	MTPJ adduction

---

[72] Vanore et al, Diagnosis and Treatment of First Metatarsophalangeal Joint Disorders. Section 2: Hallux Rigidus, Journal of Foot and Ankle Surgery 2003, 42; 3:124-36

Type 2	MTPJ adduction + IPJ flexion
Type 3	Complex multiplane

XR:
- Negative HAA, absent fibular sesamoid, negative IMA, medial subluxation of tibial sesamoid, DJD, long 1st MT

TX: postoperative splinting, shoe modification

Surgical[73]:
- loosening of the medial capsule
- reverse Austin
- tibial sesamoidectomy
- EHL transfer to plantar lateral proximal phalanx
- correct IMA
- fuse 1st MTPJ

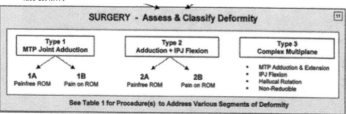

TABLE 1 Surgical options: hallux varus

Surgical Procedure (Reference)	Type 1		Type 2		Type 3
	1A	1B	2A	2B	
Percutaneous K-wire	+				
Joint release and repair (13,36)	++	+	++	+	+
Abductor hallucis release (37,38)	++	+	++	+	+
EHL transfer (Johnson) (12,13,24,39,40)					++
EHL lengthening (35)					++
Jones suspension			+	+	+
Excision tibial sesamoid (12,35)	+	+	+	+	+
IPJ arthrodesis/arthroplasty (13,41)					++
Phalangeal osteotomy (42)	+	+	+	+	
Metatarsal osteotomy (43)	+	+	+	+	+
Resection arthroplasty		++		++	
Hinge toe implant (44)		++		++	
MTP joint arthrodesis (9,13,14,45)		++		++	++

NOTE. +, appropriate; ++, ideal surgical procedure.
Abbreviations: EHL, extensor hallucis longus; K-wire, Kirschner wire.

Sesamoid fracture, sesamoiditis

ET: falls, forced DF, repetitive stress, PF 1st ray, excessive STJ pronation with 1st ray DF and eversion, equinus, rigid cavus
EP: tibial sesamoid > fibular sesamoid
CP: pain worsened by passive DF, ambulation, running, sesamoiditis
- Ilfeld's disease-agenesis of fibular sesamoid
DX: make sure to R/O bipartite sesamoids!
XR: sharp, serrated, irregular edges (bipartite sesamoids have smoother, rounder edges)
TX:
Conservative
- Activity modification, immobilization in a cast, orthotics, DANCER PAD, splints to limit DF, anti-inflammatory meds

[73] Vanore et al, Diagnosis and Treatment of First Metatarsophalangeal Joint Disorders. Section 2: Hallux Rigidus, Journal of Foot and Ankle Surgery 2003, 42; 3:124-36

Surgical
1) ORIF—prolonged return to activity
2) Sesamoidectomy—earlier return to activity (12 weeks), immediate WB
   a. Complications: hallux malleus, cocked up big toe, HAV
   b. Tibial sesamoidectomy-low risk of HAV (Canales et al, JFAS 2015[74])

Turf Toe
ET:
- Axial load to a foot in fixed equinus —> hyperextension of 1st MTPJ, disruption of plantar capsular ligamentous structure
- **Sand toe:** hyperflexion

CP: 1st MTPJ pain, restricted ROM, edema, ecchymosis

Jahss classification for trauma to 1st MTPJ

Classification	Joint	intersesamoid ligament	Treatment
1	dislocation	intact	open reduction (due to interposition of conjoined ligament)
2A	dislocation	rupture	closed reduction
2B	dislocation + sesamoid fracture	rupture	closed reduction
2C	dislocation + conjoined ligament tear	rupture	

Grading of Turf Toe

Grade	Description
Grade 1	Stretching of capsular complex
Grade 2	Partial tear
Grade 3	Frank tear

TX:
Conservative:
- Rice, strapping/splinting
Surgical:
- Sesamoidectomy (partial) better than complete due to preservation of FHB slip, function of 1st MTPJ

Forefoot Pathology

Digital contractures, hammertoe, (HT), claw toe, mallet toe, hallux malleus, flail toe, overlapping toe
- Normally, long flexors and extensors stabilized by lumbricals
- all digital contractures a result of imbalance at MTPJ
ET/RF:

---

[74] Canales, Michael B., et al. "Fact or Fiction? Iatrogenic Hallux Abducto Valgus Secondary to Tibial Sesamoidectomy." The Journal of Foot and Ankle Surgery 54.1 (2015): 82-88

Deformity	Mechanism	Phase of Gait
Flexor Stabilization	Failure of PTT to resupinate the foot results in overpronation Extrinsics (FHL/FDL) fire earlier/longer/stronger to grasp ground during midstance, overpowering the intrinsics. Digits buckle MT head pushed plantarly	Midstance
Extensor Substitution	Weak anterior muscles, EDL/EHL overpowers intrinsics during swing phase of gait, Cavus foot-EDL in position to overpower lumbricals just by passive stretch Equinus-extensors overworked to prevent tripping on forefoot	Swing
Flexor Substitution	Supinated foot with weak posterior muscles unable to PF foot during propulsion. PT, FHL, FDL overpower lumbricals.	Propulsion

1) <u>Traumatic</u>: Plantar plate rupture (predislocation syndrome), elevated compartment pressure s/p trauma/calcaneal fracture (Volkman's contractures)
2) <u>Structural</u>: cavus foot, MT length abnormality (esp for isolated 2nd digit HT 2/2 to long 2nd MT), hypermobile first ray
3) <u>Pathological</u>: Charcot-Marie-Tooth disease, muscular dystrophies
4) Shoegear-small toe box
5) <u>Congenital</u>: overlapping 5th toe

EP: Most common 2nd digit
NH:
CP:
- <u>Heloma molle</u> @ 4th interspace 2/2 to curly toe at 5th digit
  - o   head of 5th proximal phalanx rubs against base of 4th proximal phalanx
- <u>Heloma durum</u> @ dorsal IPJ
- <u>Lister's corn</u> @ lateral nail fold
- Pain confused with neuroma
- <u>TRANSVERSE PLANE</u> **congruous, deviated, or subluxed,** @ MTPJ
  - o   based on intersection of lines drawn along articular surface
- Flexibility: flexible, rigid, semi-rigid.
  - o   Reducibility determined by Kalikien push up test (pressing upwards on MT heads)
- Adductovarus deformity of the lesser digits
- Overlapping/underlapping 5th digit

DX:
1) <u>(Modified) Lachman test/dorsal/vertical stress test/drawer test/Coughlin test:</u>
   a.   With MT head immobilized and prox phalanx DF'ed, translate proximal phalanx in dorsal direction
   b.   POSITIVE TEST: >2mm or >50% dorsal displacement
2)   Kelikian pushup test
XR: gun barrel sign, look for bony changes, dislocation
TX:
Conservative:
   •   Aperture pad, crest pad, MT pad, taping/strapping, shoe adjustments, orthotics to control overpronation, Budin splint, AFO, :
Surgery:
1)   Sequential release of MTPJ (several variations):
   a.   Arthroplasty (prox phalanx head)
   b.   Extensor tenotomy
   c.   Extensor hood release
   d.   Extensor T lengthening
   e.   Flexor T transfer
2)   Overlapping 5th toe:
   a.   Incision from DISTAL MEDIAL TO PROXIMAL LATERAL
   b.   Z plasty or V-Y plasty

c. Z tendon lengthening

Soft tissue procedures

Procedure	Description
(Flexor or extensor) percutaneous tenotomy	**for hammertoe:** cut @ PIPJ (release FDL/FDB) **for clawtoe:** cut @ DIPJ (release FDL)
Extensor tendon lengthening, Z-lengthening	proximal to MPJ more for extensor induced HT add to arthroplasty or arthrodesis procedure
Capsulotomy	PIPJ or MPJ Includes extensor hood release, J maneuver to release collaterals can use McGlamry elevator
Flexor tendon transfer	dorsal transfer of FDL to help "bring down" digit **Girdlestone Taylor:** bisect tendon, flexor re-attached dorsally and sutured together to make a sling over proximal phalanx **Kuwada/Dockery:** re-route tendon through DISTAL drill hole **Schuberth:** re-route tendon through PROXIMAL drill hole

5th digit procedures*

Procedure	Description
Derotational arthoplasty	For adductovarus 5th digit: 1) PIPJ arthroplasty 2) oblique removal of skin
Medial MTPJ capsulotomy	
V-Y skin platy	
Ruiz Mora procedure	USE: congenital overlapping 5th toe Total phalangectomy of the proximal phalanx. SE: risk flail toe due to excessive removal of bone
Syndactyly	fuse one digit to a normal adjacent digit to "bring down" Good treatment for flail toe SE: invagination of skin edges, extension/flexion deformity
Condylectomy	
Z-plasty of skin	

*Correction of 5th toe deformity can result in increases pressure in 4th digit —> 4th HT

Type of procedure	Indications	Technique	Complication
Arthroplasty	for FLEXOR induced HT- shortens distance for FDL to pull	**Resectional** (Keller) **Interpositional**-interposition of tissue to keep inflammatory surfaces apart **Implant**	**Recurrence** at PIPJ (esp 2nd) **Flail toe** (overshortened toe) **Unstable MTPJ** **Hemosiderin** deposit

Type of procedure	Indications	Technique	Complication
Arthrodesis	Rigidity Recurence Transverse plane Dislocation Central digits	-Add PIPJ arthroplasty -Fuse proximal phalanx in 5-10 deg DF -K wire (0.045, 0.054, or 0.062), peg-in-hole -K-wire through proximal phalanx or distal 1/3 of MT -retrograde drilling from base of middle phalanx distally, then drive through proximal phalanx -K wire left in for 6 weeks	**Transverse** MTPJ deformity **"Overloading syndrome"**-ulceration, stress fx at 2nd MT head **K wire SE:** bend, break, interruption of cartilage, lack of compression, migration of wire, pin tract infection
Implant arthroplasty	-Does not shorten PIPJ	-Corrects transverse plane deformity (Sung)	
Amputation	-For elderly		

Metatarsalgia
ET: Neuroma, plantar plate rupture, stress fracture, abnormal MT parabola, foreign body, soft tissue mass, bone tumor, epidermal inclusion cyst, AVN, predislocation syndrome,
MT parabola
- Articulated: 2>3>1>4>5
- Disarticulated: 2>3>5>4>1

CP:

Symptom	Diagnosis
Decreased ROM/crepitus	Osseus
Hyperextended MPJ, pain with palpation of MPJ	Plantar plate/collateral ligament rupture

DX: radiograph, MRI, CT, US (soft tissue), radionucleotide scanning, arthrography
TX:

Predislocation syndrome, 2nd MPJ instability, plantar plate dysfunction, plantar plate rupture, mono-articular nontraumatic synovitis, crossover second toe deformity, metatarsus proximus, splay toe
Trauma OR Chronic microtrauma —> chronic inflammation of 2nd MTPJ—> rupture of plantar plate (or capsule, collateral ligaments)

ET/RF:
- **Anatomy of plantar plate**-"crimp morphology", Chinese fingertrap
- **Trauma**
- **Chronic microtrauma**
  - MOST COMMON ETIOLOGY: elongated MT or short neighboring MT
  - Chronic inflammation-capsulitis/bursitis/synovitis
  - Rupture of lateral collateral ligament/damage to MTPJ joint capsule —>rupture of plantar plate
- Biomechanics:
  - Because flexor tendon sheath/plantar plate directly under 2nd MTPJ (offset medially for others)
- Anatomy
  - Long 2nd MT
  - PF'ed MT
  - Hypermobile 1st ray
  - Short adjacent ray

- o   MT adductus: close apposition of MT heads
- Concomittant HAV deformity:
  - o   increased transfer force to 2nd MT
  - o   medial pull of hallux sesamoids causes 2nd digit to drift medially
- Shoegear-high heels
- Increased age
- Arthropathy
  - o   Freiberg's infraction
  - o   Synovitis/bursitis
  - o   **Inflammatory arthropathy**-rheumatoid, Reiters, psoriatic

EP: women >> men

NH:
- Plantar plate serves as stabilizer during WB
- Plantar plate has poor healing capability
- **Progressive deformity**-surgery ONLY DEFINITIVE treatment

CP:
- "Grape-like" swelling, like a stone bruise on the ball of the foot.
- **Painful MT head /callus**
- **Crossover toe**: rupture of lateral collateral and suspensory ligament
- **Hammertoe**: rupture of plantar plate
- Painful upon palpation and range of motion, especially PF
- PIPJ contracture

DX:

PREDISLOCATION SYNDROME IS A CLINICAL DIAGNOSIS
- (Modified) Lachman test/dorsal/vertical stress test/drawer test/Coughlin test
- Plantar plate ruptures can go undiagnosed
- Visual inspection of plantar plate during Weil osteotomy

Arthrogram
- Plantar plate/capsule TEAR* —> DORSAL injection results in leakage of dye into <u>FLEXOR</u> tendon sheath
- *partial tear would not result in leakage
- Could be false positive if leaks nearby—bursa formation, NOT a plantar plate rupture.

MRI-useful to make surgical decisions
- helps distinguish between partial and full tear of plantar plate
- helps ID collateral ligament tear

Ultrasound

TX:

Clinical presentation	Treatment
no instability	
subluxable	plantar plate repair + HT repair +/- FDL transfer/osteotomy
dislocatable	arthroplasty/arthrodesis/amputation
dislocated	arthroplasty/arthrodesis/amputation

- Correct 1st MTPJ pathology if present, as 2nd digit follows 1st digit

Conservative: (symptomatic relief)
- Conservative tx NEVER heals the pathology (avascular fibrocartilage)
- Offloading, splinting, orthoses, rocker-bottom shoes, **MT pad**, Budin splint, crest pad, NSAIDs, corticosteroid injection
- **Spica taping**

Surgical:

Ligamentous
- Flexor tendon transfer: (original) GOLD STANDARD
  - o   good for transverse plane deformity
  - o   DYNAMIC tethering

- Capsulotomy or capsulorraphy
- Plantar plate repair: using plantar aponeurosis, FDL
  - Dorsal vs plantar approach
    - ☐ Dorsal-complete resection of plantar plate and re-attachment
    - ☐ Plantar-direct visualization of plantar plate
  - Restores normal anatomy
  - Stability to MTPJ
  - STATIC stability
  - adddresses pain 2/2 MT head herniation
  - NOT good for deformity at IPJ
- Extensor tendon lengthening
- EDB tendon transfer
- Reefing of plantar lateral capsule, collateral ligament repair, MTPJ capsule repair

Osseus

- IPJ arthrodesis (K-wire or implant)
- Arthroplasty/arthrodesis
  - TRANSVERSE plane correction
- Lesser MTPJ arthrodesis
  - Mostly for 2nd MTPJ
  - Add PIPJ arthroplasty
- Fuse proximal phalanx in 5-10 degrees DF
  - Risk: "overloading syndrome"—ulceration and stress fracture at MT head

Distal MT	
Weil	**Indications**: long, PF, or angular deformed MT
	- Good for TRANSVERSE plane deformity 2/2 long 2nd MT, to take pressure off intrinsic tendons
	- Does NOT stabilize MTPJ, just decreases pressure sub MTPJ
	Technique:
	- DORSAL DISTAL —> PLANTAR PROXIMAL
	Pearls:
	- VISUALIZE PLANTAR PLATE for tears
	- Don't PF the MT head
	Complications:
	- Transfer lesions
	- Recurrence
	- **Floating toe/flail toe-**
	- Toes normally passively PF due to windlass. Shortening of MT leads to reduced tension in flexors, plantar fascia, and "dampens" the windlass mechanism (Christensen)
	- could be 2/2 to ruptured plantar plate
	- **Dorsal contracture**-prevent by placing pin in MTPJ to keep flexor tendon in tension
Weil + Plantar plate repair	reduces risk of floating toe 2/2 to ruptured plantar plate
Jacoby	V-osteotomy, can PF or DF
Duvries	plantar condylectomy on both sides of MPJ
Chevron	Jacoby with removal of bone to shorten MT
DFWO	same as Waterman

MT shaft	
cylindrical shortening	
Giannestras step-down	Z-shaped cut to shorten and DF MT
MT Base	
DFWO	1mm dorsal shortening = 10 deg DF
Buckholtz	oblique DF wedge

Capsulitis

ET:
- Mechanical: plantar plate tear
- Arthritic: RA, seronegative arthridities

TX:
Conservative:
- Offloading, NSAIDs, corticosteroid injection
- Oral steroids: Medrol dosepack

Surgical
- Synovectomy
- Repair of plantar plate tear
- Arthroplasty, chondroplasty

Stress fracture

ET: repetitive normal cyclic loading on bone, microtrauma,
RF: bone mineral deficiency (vit D deficiency), dancers, inflammatory arthropathy, osteoporosis, joint deformity, chronic steroids
EP: females >> males
DX:
- Clinical exam: tuning fork
- Radiograph:
  - Bony callus may not develop for 2-3 weeks (30-50% de-mineralization needed)
  - Healing bone callus
- Bone scan: positive uptake
- Labs: Ca^{2+}, phos, all phos, vit D
CP: most common: $2^{nd}/3^{rd}$ MT neck
TX: offload, walking boot, surgical shoe

Arthridities

***prior to surgery, obtain C-spine XR due to unstable vertebral bodies which may compress spinal cord

Osteoarthritis, osteoarthrosis, degenerative joint disease (DJD)
Deterioration of cartilage—>exposure of subchondral bone —> subchondral sclerosis—> eburnation—>osteophyte

ET:
- Primary OA-idiopathic
- Secondary OA (degenerative joint disease)-repetitive strain

NH:
- Eburnation: *degeneration* of cartilage, subchondral bone exposed

CP:
- ASYMMETRICAL non-inflammatory arthritis

- Morning stiffness <1 hour (vs RA >1 hour)
- Deep achy pain worse with activity, prolonged standing and activity
- Thickening of subchondral bone
- Heberden's nodes: enlargement of DIPJ
- Bouchard's nodes: enlargement at PIPJ

PE: decreased ROM, crepitus

Radiograph:
- Joint space narrowing
- Subchondral sclerosis (thickening)
- Osteophyte (dorsal flag) aka detritus aka loose body aka "joint mice",

TX:
- Oral: NSAIDs—ibuprofen,
  - If GI history: celebrex (caution cardiac abnorm), tramadol
- Injections:
  - Steroid
  - Hyaluronic acid (Euflexxa, 1% sodium hyaluronate)
  - Bracing:
  - Rocker bottom shoe
  - lace up ankle brace (frontal plane) + CAM boot (saggital plane)
  - OA is the only arthritis treatable with surgery

Rheumatoid arthritis

NH:
- Insidious onset
  - Synovial fibroblast snyoviocytes (SFS) become autoimmune
  - Cytokine/chemokine inflammation
  - Chronic synovitis
  - Joint destruction targeting articular cartilage, collateral ligaments, tendon, bone

EP: 0.8%, females > males

RF: HLA, CTLA4 gene

CP:

Natural history: monocyclic or polycyclic

General:
- **Felty's syndrome**: RA + neutropenia, splenomegaly, hyperpigmentation
  - possible low grade fever, fatigue, weight loss, malaise
- immunocompromised 2/2 DMARDs—inc risk tuberculosis
- influenza and pneumococcal vaccines are SAFE

MSK
- **Mostly in 4th/5th MTPJ of foot**
- Ulnar (!lateral) deviation of toes, pes planus, HAV deformity 2/2 to synovitis
- SYMMETRICAL, inflammatory arthritis, joint pain, redness, warmth
- Subluxation of MTPJ
- Morning stiffness for 1-2 hours, better with motion, progressively more painful throughout the day
- Cervical spine involvement
- Gel phenomenon-pain worst after rest
- Pannus-synovial expansion of macrophage, osteoclast, snyovial fibroblast, lymphocytes that destroy articular cartilage
- Anterior shift of forefoot fat pad
- Rheumatoid nodules-SC painless nodules over bony prominence found in 25%
- Baker's cyst-synovial fluid cyst in popliteal fossa
- Felty's syndrome-RA with splenomegaly, pigmented spots in LE
- Swan neck deformity: hyperextension of PIPJ, DIPJ flexion
- Boutonniere deformity: flexion of PIPJ, DIPJ hyperextension (same as hammertoe)
  - Ulceration 2/2 NEUROPATHY + DEFORMITY, increased ABI, corticosteroid use (tissue fragility, poor wound healing), reduced self care 2/2 to poor dexterity, rheumatoid nodules

DX:

LABS:
- Rheumatoid panel (ANA, RF, ESR)
- Anti-CCP

- ACPA (Anti citrullinated protein antibody)
- ANA positive
- + RF labs
- Elevated PMN

Criteria for diagnosis of RA

Guidelines for classification	Criteria
4/7 required for diagnosis	morning stiffness lasting at least 1 hr before improvement
patient with 2+ clinical diagnoses are NOT excluded	arthritis of 3+ of the 14 joint areas
symptoms present for > 6 wks	arthritis of the hand joints
	rheumatoid nodules
	positive serum RF
	radiologic changes

TX:
Lower extremity: orthotics
Medical:
- ASA, corticosteroids, antimalarials, DMARDS
- Infliximab-increased postoperative infection 2/2 DMARD/TNF alpha inhibitors (especially when taking <1 drug)
- Methotrexate: MOA: folic acid antagonist, used in chemotherapy
    o SE include GI upset, stomatitis
- Plaquenil (hydrochloroquine)-anti-malarial
- Chloroquine, minocycline, cyclosporine, adalimumab, etanercept
- glucocorticoids
Conservative: orthopedic shoes, orthoses, padding
Surgical:
Joint destructive
- Hoffman-MT heads 2-5 resected (pan MT head resection) + 1st MTPJ fusion
    o Leave about 1cm gap (tip of index finger) in the joint
    o Monitor circulatory status of the toes post-operatively
    o #1 SE: recurrent plantar IPK
- Gocht-prox phalanx base resection
- Clayton-MT heads and prox phalanx base resection
- MT head resection, MTPJ fusion
- Keller
Joint preserving
- Scarf + Weil/shortening MT osteotomy-joint preserving procedure
- synovectomy

Synovial Fluid Analysis

	normal	OA	RA	septic	gout	hemorrhagic
color	straw			green		red
viscosity	high	high	low		low	

	normal	OA	RA	septic	gout	hemorrhagic
clarity	transparent	transp.		opaque		bloody
crystal					yes	
WBC	<200	200-2k	2k-10k	2k-100k	2k-40k	200-2k
gram stain				positive		

Gout
- **Primary gout**-metabolic disorder
- **Secondary gout**-acquired, medicine induced

Primary Gout	Overproducer (10%)	Undersecreter (90%)
Diagnosis	metabolic gout	renal gout
Uric acid (blood and urine)	elevated uric acid	low/normal uric acid
Etiology	genetic enzyme defect	kidney problem
Treatment	allopurinol	probenecid

ET/RF:
- elevated uric acid levels
- De novo pathway vs salvage pathway
- Age, obesity
- Purine-rich foods (alcohol, seafood, red meats)
- NOT always elevated uric acid because *may have resolved* since acute gouty attack

EP: men >> women. NEVER in pre-menopausal women (estrogen increases uric acid excretion)

CP:
- 1st MTPJ (podagra)
    - O   predilection for foot due to: low temperature (poor urate solubility), low pH
- Dactylitis-"sausage toe", red, hot, swollen, joint
- Tophi-chalky deposits at other joints-elbows, hands
    - O   risk for ulceration or sinus tract
- Recurrent "attacks" over the past couple of months
- History of CKD, kidney stones

4 stages (**usually resolves in 1 week**):
1. Asymptomatic hyperuricemia
2. Acute gout
3. Intercritical gout
4. Chronic tophaceous gout

DX: Needle aspiration
- Still beneficial to tap if no fluid present
- Culture
- Polarized light microscopy
    - O   Monosodium urate crystals (negative birefringent needle shape)
    - O   YELLOW when parallel to lens, BLUE when perpendicular to lens
- Martini sign-needle through macrophage
- Gram stain
- Uric acid level from 24 hour urine collection
    - O   <600mg: undersecretor

o   >600mg: overproducer

TX:
- Diet
- Medical treatment:
  - Allopurinol 100mg ("pick ax" for uric acid crystal, chronic treatment,) + 0.5mg colchicine (anti-inflammatory, acute gouty attacks)
    o   Acute attack:
      1) **NSAID** (indomethacin 50mg TID or naproxen 500mg BID) x 5-7 days
      2) **Colchicine**: for NSAID intolerance
      3) **Steroids**: intra-articular steroid injection, prednisone
      4) **IL-1 inhibitor**
    *Do NOT use ASA, which will decrease uric acid secretion
- Surgical treatment
- I&D washout, arthroplasty, arthrodesis

Gout medication

Drug	Dose	MOA/SE	Use
Colchicine	0.5-1mg QD/BID x1 wk til pain gone or N/V/D Reduce by 50% in renal/hepatic dysfcn/ elderly	**inhibit neutrophil from phagocytosing urate crystals** ==> anti-inflammatory SE: N/V/D, weakness, neuropathy	Acute
Allopurinol	300mg QD Labs (LFT, uric acid 3 wks after start)	Uricostatic, **inhibit xanthine oxidase** & the prod of uric acid SE: rare Steven Johnson	Chronic, Overprod of uric acid
Uloric (febuxostat)		**xanthine oxidase inhibitor**	
Probenecid	250mg BID, increase dose	Uricosuric outcompetes, prevents reabsorption of uric acid at proximal tubule (**P**robenecid = **P**roximal tubule) SE: kidney stones	Chronic, Undersecret of uric acid
Indomethacin	25-50mg TID	strong NSAID COX inhibitor, SE: inhibit cartilage formation, renal	Acute
Naproxen	500mg BID	NSAID	Acute

Pseudogout, calcium pyrophosphate dihydrate (CPPD), chondrocalcinosis
EP: older women > 80
CP: longer course than gout

Juvenile Rheumatoid arthritis, juvenile RA, JRA, juvenile idiopathic arthritis
ET: unknown,
EP: <16 y.o., 90% present with foot problem
CP:
- Systemic (Still's disease)—joint pain, fevers, rash, uveitis
- Predilection for large joints
- Fusion of C2-C4
- Polyarticular JRA—large and small joints
- Pauciarticular JRA—only a few joints
Labs:
- RF often negative
- Juvenile arthritis foot disability index (JAFI)

Seronegative arthridities AKA spondylarthropathies

Seronegative = absence of positive RF

Seronegative Arthridities	Description
	ET: link to HLA-B27 EP: Male >> Female CP: ▫ Enthesitis: inflammation at tendinous insertions: Achilles tendinitis or plantar fasciitis ▫ Dactylitis AKA sausage digit TX: TNF alpha inhibitors
Ankylosing spondylitis (AS)	CP: Lumbar pain, very stiff, inflexible backbone, sacroillitis, limitation of chest expansion, hip arthritis, neck pain, kyphosis, **poker spine**-stiff, inflexible, aortic insufficiency DX: Schoeber's test-ability of patient to flex lower back, **XR:** "bamboo spine" — spine fusion
Diffuse idiopathic skeletal hyperostosis (DISH), Forrester's disease	similar to AS except no sacroilitis huge sharp, well defined calcaneal bone spur
Psoriatic arthritis	• Seen with psoriasis skin disease, oily pitting nail changes • Morning stiffness • **Pencil-in-cup** whittling • **Salmon-pink** papule • psoriasis vulgaris-silver plaque • psoriasis pustulosis-pustules and vesicles
Reiter's syndrome/ reactive arthritis	ET: Triggered by infectious agent outside joint: 1) STD (chlamydia) 2) GI/dysenteric CP: **Triad:** can't see can't pee can't climb a tree (arthritis, urethritis, conjunctivitis) • **Lover's heel**-fluffy, wooly heel spur • Stomatitis • Can't climb a tree with skin like this either (Keratoderma blennorrhagicum):
Inflammatory bowel (IBD) Crohn's, Ulcerative Colitis	Arthritic flares parallel bowel disease
Systemic Lupus erythematosus (SLE)	*multi systemic disease of connective tissue* ET: can be drug induced CP: VASCULITIS (2/2 immunoglobulin deposits), arthralgia (lack of erosion), butterfly rash, photosensitivity, nephritis, Black women DX: + ANA, **+anti dsDNA** TX: anti-malarials

Arthridities

	Etiology	Details

Septic arthritis	bacterial	Subchondral resorption Osteolysis "bone destruction" (7-10 days) Joint space widening >50k WBC
Neuropathic osteoarthropathy (Charcot)		Subchondral resorption Subluxation/dislocation Arthritis mutilans Detritus (loose bodies)
Osteoarthritis, post-traumatic	non inflammatory	Asymmetrical joint space narrowing Osteophyte (2/2 chronic inflammation to bring in fibroblast) Subchondral sclerosis, EBURNATION (increased density, thickening of subchondral bone 2/2 to increased inflammation) Subchondral cyst (fluid-filled sac from extrusion of hyaluronic acid) **Medial** MT head erosion Detritus (loose bodies), joint mice
Rheumatoid arthritis	inflammatory	(Symmetrical) fibular deviation MEDIAL erosion except 5th MPJ (lipping/beaking/flagging) Polyarticular Subchondral osteopenia NO erosion of IPJ of lesser digits (EVEN) joint space narrowing no new bone formation Pseudocyst (bone loss) Dot-dash "skip" pattern Hand, wrist, cervical spine (anasthesia caution!) Early joint space widening, late joitn space narrowing (ankylosis)
Psoriatic arthritis (Seronegative arthropathy) (similar to RA)	inflammatory	Medial + LATERAL erosion of MTPJ, IPJ **Arthritis mutilans: medial and lateral** MT head erosion ("pencil in cup")-obliteration of the joint Whittling Joint space widening due to subchondral resorption (half of phalanx missing) Whiskering/ivory phalanx (increased density) of distal hallux phalanx Periostitis
Gout	inflammatory	C-shaped erosion, well defined Periarticular (extra-articular) = NORMAL joint space Soft tissue calcification next to joint space Martel's sign—"rat bite" overhanging margin Tophi in soft tissue 1st MTPJ, hallux IPJ Monoarticular
Pseudogout, CPPD (calcium pyrophosphate dihydrate deposition), chondrocalcinosis	inflammatory	Tendon/bursal/joint capsule calcification TN joint, knee, wrist

HADD (calcium hydroxyapatite deposition disease)	non inflammatory	Soft tissue calcification Shoulder
PVNS (pigmented villonodular synovitis)	non inflammatory	Soft tissue tumor causes pressure atrophy of adjacent bones C-shaped erosions

Septic Arthritis, septic joint,

SURGICAL EMERGENCY: NEED TO RULE OUT FOR ANY ACUTE MONO-ARTICULAR ARTHRITIS

ET:
- Hematogenous seeding (most common)
- Direct inoculation
- Extension from adjacent infection
- Cartilage damage by bacterial enterotoxins and indirectly from the host immune response to bacteria

RF: DM, implant, IVDU RA, OA, immunosuppression, crystal arthropathy, cutaneous ulcers

CP: ABRUPT red, hot swollen joint.
- Fever, systemic illness is NOT necessary
- Knee (MC), hip, ankle
- Pseudoparalysis of limb especially in young children

DX: Joint aspiration : positive gram stain OR positive cultures
- Try to avoid area of cellulitis
- positive gram stain, synovial fluid culture, high nucleated cell count >50 x 10^9 cells/L CRP/ESR, WBC > 50k
- MOST COMMON:
    o   Adults: Staph aureus
    o   Children: GBS
    o   Sexually active <30 y.o. N. gonorrhea
- a type of migratory arthritis

TX:
- SURGICAL EMERGENCY to prevent irreversible cartilage damage: Emergent surgical I&D
- Daily drainage of purulent material from joint via aspiration
    o   History of inflammatory arthropathy, large joint, S. aureus infection, or hx DM increase failure of single surgical debridement[75]
    o   Course of IV antibiotics based on culture results
    o   Delayed treatment results in joint degeneration, osteonecrosis, or joint instability

Scleroderma, systemic sclerosis

Systemic disorder of connective tissue and fibrosis of organs. Sclerosis, hardening of the skin

CP:
- **CREST**: calcinosis, Raynaud's esophageal dysfunction, sclerodactyly, telangiectasia
- Mouse-face-induration/thickening/tightening of skin

ET: females >> males

Dermatomyositis/polymyositis
- Polymyositis-weakness of limb girdles
- Dermatomyositis-Gottron's papules, flat papules over dorsal knuckles
- Both-heliotrope rash (pink purple), facial lesions

Sjogren's syndrome

ET: Decreased secretion of exocrine gland, enlarged parotic

CP:

Keratoconjunctivitis sicca-dry eyes

---

[75] Hunter, Joshua G., et al. "Risk Factors for Failure of a Single Surgical Debridement in Adults with Acute Septic Arthritis." The Journal of Bone & Joint Surgery 97.7 (2015): 558-564.

Xerostomia-dry mouth
DX: **Schirmer's test**-litmus paper to eye, positive test if >5mm

Pes Planus & Associated Conditions

PTTD (posterior tibial tendon dysfunction) aka posterior tibial tendon insufficiency (PTTI) aka Adult acquired flatfoot, Pes planus, pes planovalgus, pes valgus, adult acquired flatfoot deformity (AAFD), flexible flatfoot, collapsing pes planovalgus
FAILURE OF INTRINSIC/EXTRINSIC/DYNAMIC STABILIZERS OF FOOT
more than an inflammatory condition or tendon rupture, but MUSCLE IMBALANCE

Questions to ask: skeletal maturity, uni/bilateral, flexible/rigid, symptomatic?

ET/NH:

Which came first? PTTD or arch collapse/hindfoot valgus?

1) **PTT is #1 dynamic arch support**
    a. contracts during stance and mid stance to slow STJ pronation
2) Overworked PTT ==> chronic insufficiency/tendinosis
3) PTT failure
4) Rupture, attenuation of PTT *PLUS static supporting structures of medial hindfoot (spring ligament (81%), deltoid ligament, plantar fascia (#1 arch support), long/short plantar ligaments)*
5) Inability for MTJ to lock to form rigid lever
6) Collapse of the medial arch, transverse plane deformity—>increases strain on PTT
7) Peroneals fire unopposed
8) Hindfoot valgus, forefoot abductus
9) Gastroc-soleus now pulls on TN joint, not first MT heads.
    a. **Equinus**
        i. Foot compensates for lack of ankle DF by pronating at STJ and MTJ
        ii. Excessive forefoot pressure causes instability of peroneus longus, hypermobile 1st ray, overpronation
        iii. Orthotics in the presence of equinus will not work!!! Results in metatarsalgia/arch pain
    b. Ligamentous laxity (spring ligament, deltoid, interosseus talocalcaneal ligament, plantar aponeurosis, long/short plantar)
    c. Suprapedal structural deformities
        i. Limb length difference (long leg causes pronation)
        ii. Coxa valgum (outward angulation of femoral shaft)
        iii. Genu varum/valgum
        iv. Femoral retroversion (external rotation of femur)
        v. External tibial torsion
        vi. Blount's disease (medial tibia osteochondrosis leading to bow-leggedness)
    d. Biomechanical deformity (structural or positional)
        i. Lateral column instability more severe than medial column instability
        ii. **Most commonly FF varus, RF valgus**
        iii. FF varus (osseus)
        iv. FF supinatus (soft tissue)
        v. Flexible FF valgus
        vi. RF valgus/varus
        vii. Abducted FF
        viii. Externally rotated hindfoot
    e. Neuromuscular imbalance (polio, CP)

RF: obesity, DM, HTN, steroid exposure, accessory navicular, Ehler Danlos
EP: Adults only, females > 50 y.o., obesity, diseases resulting in tendon degeneration

Types of flatfoot

Flexible	Rigid	Flexible AND Rigid
Congenital calcaneovalgus	CVT	PTTD (early vs late)
Kidner foot	Tarsal coalition	MT adductus
	RA	

Forefoot biomechanical pathology

	Forefoot varus	Forefoot supinatus
Source	Osseus (structural deformity)	Soft tissue (compensatory), seen in PTTD
Reducibility with STJ neutral	Nonreducible	Reducible
Effect on flatfoot	Induces STJ pronation	Created by STJ pronation
Occurrence	Less common	More common**
Treatment		Lapidus, Hoke, Cotton
Planes affected	Frontal	Triplanar
Part of foot affected	Forefoot	MTJ

CP:
- Medial malleolar or medial arch pain at insertion of PT
  - o PTT rupture-most commonly posterior to medial malleolus (avascularity)
- Acutely painful foot with history of pop or snap
- PF, internally rotated talus
- Abducted, supinated/varus FF, RF valgus
  - o External hip rotation
  - o Internally rotated tibia (anteriorly displaced fibula)
- Arch pain 2/2 to overworked abductor hallucis
- Metatarsalgia, plantar fasciitis, postural symptoms, back pain, inability to stand for long periods of time, difficulty walking/running,
- TRIAD (same as tarsal coalition): Achy pain at sinus tarsi/STJ, limited ROM, peroneal spasm
- shin splints 2/2 overpronation

Johnson and Strom classification[76] with Myerson[77] modification:

	Stage 1	Stage 2 (most common)	Stage 3	Stage 4 (Myerson)
Tendon condition	Tenosynovitis	partial rupture/split tears, ELONGATION	tendon rupture	deltoid ligament degeneration
Rearfoot	No deformity	FLEXIBLE deformity	RIGID deformity, STJ arthritis	ANKLE valgus
Examination	No deformity	weak heel rise, + too many toes	no heel rise	valgus talus
Surgical treatment	soft tissue	soft tissue + osteotomy	osteotomy + fusion	fusion
Complaint	pain at insertion	pain along PT course	lateral hindfoot pain	generalized hindfoot pain

[76] JOHNSON, KENNETH A., and DAVID E. STROM. "Tibialis posterior tendon dysfunction." Clinical orthopaedics and related research 239 (1989): 196-206.
[77] Bluman, Eric M., Craig I. Title, and Mark S. Myerson. "Posterior tibial tendon rupture: a refined classification system." Foot and ankle clinics 12.2 (2007): 233-249

ACFAS Modification[78]

| Stage 2A | Early | Minimal hindfoot valgus, <30% TN uncovering |
| Stage 2B | Late | Moderate to severe hindfoot valgus, >30% TN uncovering |

EXAM:
- Talar head prominence, calcaneal eversion
- Palpate along PT tendon proximally to insertion
- PTT mm strength: put finger on 1st MT head with pt PF, max everted
- "Too many toes sign"-check for FF abduction
- FLEXIBLE VS. RIGID
  - o "Single/double heel rise test"-holding wall for support,
    - reducibility of valgus heel to varus
    - re-creation of medial arch
  - o "Hubscher maneuver"/Jack's test/Toe Test of Jack-while WB, DF of hallux to look for arch/functional Windlass mechanism
    - Positive-flexible, negative-rigid, osseus restriction

DX:
- XR
  - o CORA: lateral NCJ (early), TN (late) fault
  - o Navicular looks smaller on AP view when foot pronated position

Planal dominance

Direction STJ moves towards	increased deformity in which plane?
parallel to sagittal plane	transverse plane
parallel to transverse plane	frontal plane
parallal to frontal plane	sagittal plane

Radiographic angles used to classify planal dominance[79]

Sagittal Plane	Front Plane	Transverse Plane
INC talar declination	DEC 1st MT declination	INC AP Talocalc angle
INC lateral talocalc angle	DEC height sustentaculum tali	INC Calcaneocuboid angle
DEC Calc inclination angle	INC superimposition of lateral lesser tarsus	DEC talonavicular congruency
NC breach	Widening of lesser tarsus AP view	DEC forefoot to rearfoot adduction
	Lateralized tibiocalc angle (long leg calcanea axial view)	

- US-dynamic assessment of PTT tenosynovitis, spring ligament

[78] Shibuya, Naohiro, Ryan T. Kitterman, and Daniel C. Jupiter. "Evaluation of the Rearfoot Component (Module 3) of the ACFAS Scoring Scale." The Journal of Foot and Ankle Surgery 53.5 (2014): 544-547.
[79] Labovitz, Jonathan M. "The algorithmic approach to pediatric flexible pes planovalgus." Clinics in podiatric medicine and surgery 23.1 (2006): 57-76

- MRI-check for integrity of PTT, spring ligament, interosseus talocalcaneal ligament, deltoid ligament (stage 3 deformity) edema, arthritic changes

Funk[80]/Conti[81]

Funk	intra-op appearance	Conti	MRI reading
1	tendon avulsion	1	tenosynovitis
2	missubstance rupture	2	longitudinal splits
3	in-continuity tear	3	complete rupture
4	tenosynovitis		

TX:

Conservative:
- Rest, strapping, NSAIDs, shoe modification, functional bracing (Arizona brace), orthotics, below the knee cast, weight loss, physical therapy
- PTTD: CAM boot 6-8 weeks
- Orthotics: break them in (wear for 1 hr, 2 hrs, etc)

Surgical:

> *Goal: Achieve the best correction while preserving as much of the joints and their function as possible*
> *Simulated WB intra-operatively*

SOFT TISSUE:
- POSTERIOR RELEASE
- isolated soft tissue procedures indicated only in early, flexible flatfoot
- consider bony procedure i.e. MCSO, arthroeresis to protect tendon and soft tissue procedure

Procedure	Description
Tenosynovectomy of PTT	debridement of PTT, when NO tendon rupture/tear present
Spring ligament reconstruction/reefing/desmopl asty	**Etiology:** • Spring ligament most common structure damaged in PTTD **Anatomy:** • blends with deltoid ligament • spring ligament complex: 1) superomedial 2) medial plantar oblique 3) plantar inferior (MC involved) **Indication:** • No benefits to ligament plication (Mann), hard to study the benefit of isolated procedure • repair when appears attenuated **Technique:** • pants over vest imbrication, tightening of spring ligament. • address both bands • reconstruction (allograft, TA, PB, PL) > plication
Deltoid ligament repair	

---

[80] Funk, DANIEL A., J. R. Cass, and K. A. Johnson. "Acquired adult flat foot secondary to posterior tibial-tendon pathology." The Journal of Bone & Joint Surgery 68.1 (1986): 95-102.

[81] Conti, Stephen, James Michelson, and Melvin Jahss. "Clinical significance of magnetic resonance imaging in preoperative planning for reconstruction of posterior tibial tendon ruptures." Foot & Ankle International 13.4 (1992): 208-214

Procedure	Description
Tendon transfer (FDL, FHL, PB to FDL, PB to PL tenodesis)	FDL: opposition to PB, expendable, proximity to PTT Indications: • Severely degenerated PTT • Flexible deformity • Heel rise-presence of STJ inversion • CAUTION to perform in isolation Technique: • cut FDL just proximal to Knot of Henry • Proximal tendon: tenodese to PTT, • Distal tendon: tenodese to FHL to maintain digital PF OR leave alone • consider spring ligament reefing in conjunction
Young tenosuspension	
Kidner	Not a corrective procedure, but relieves enlarged navicular tuberosity remove accessory navicular until flush with medial cuneiform, re-route PTT distal/plantar via bone anchor/through navicular
Cobb	TA split proximally, graft re-routed through medial cuneiform, tenodesed to PTT SACRIFICES major inverter/adductor of foot
TAL/gastroc recession	ALWAYS to restore CIA

SAGITTAL PLANE (medial column) procedures

Saggital plane	Type	*"young kids heave miller at the cotton lap low"*
Young tenosuspension (Keyhole)	Soft tissue	Technique: reroute TA through a "keyhole" in navicular with insertion intact, corrects TN/NC fault. PROS:Maintains inversion, DF, gives PL mechanical advantage CONS: only for flexible deformity, saggital plane
Kidner	Soft tissue	Indication: • Not a corrective procedure, but relieves enlarged navicular tuberosity Technique: • remove accessory navicular until flush with medial cuneiform, re-route PTT distal/plantar via bone anchor/through navicular
Hoke	Bony + fusion	NC(1 & 2) plantar-based CBWO, arthrodesis
Miller	Fusion	NC & FMCJ arthrodesis
Cotton, aka medial cuneiform opening wedge osteotomy (MCOW)	Bony	Technique: dorsal OBWO of medial cuneiform MOA: Corrects forefoot supinatus Pros: Stabilizes medial column, off-loads stress on lateral column, maintain first ray mobility
Lapidus	Fusion	1st MT/med cuneiform fusion

Saggital plane	Type	*"young kids heave miller at the cotton lap low"*
Lowman	ST + fusion	TN arthrodesis + reroute TA under navicular, attached to spring ligament, slip of Achilles fused to navicular + TAL
NC fusion	Fusion	
TAL/gastroc recession	Soft tissue	

TRANSVERSE PLANE

Transverse plane	

Evans aka LCL aka anterior calcaneal osteotomy	**Indication:**
	• MTJ instability
	• >40% TN uncovering
	• good procedure for stage 2 PTTD (flexible)
	• Better radiographic correction than MCSO
	Contraindication:
	• Foot with a MAA component
	Technique:
	• **Graft**: Allograft comparable to autograft, Allograft + PRP may be even better than autograft
	   o Graft 1.5 cm prox to CC joint (prevent hitting the anterior facet) Max graft size: 1 cm (expect graft to compress 20%), normally 8mm-12mm No inc CCJ pressure until graft >8cm
	   o Triangular (less CCJ pain) or trapezoidal wedge
	   o caution not to violate anterior/medial facet and sustentaculum tali
	• **Fixation**: none, percutaneous K wire, screw, plate
	   o Some can argue not necessary due to large tension force, but secures sagittal plane position. Expedites healing and diminishes nonunion risk.
	   o Plate SE: peroneal irritation
	MOA:
	• 1) RF valgus 2) FF abduction 3) raises med long arch, unloading 1st MCJ
	• reduces inversion demand on PTT, reduces Achilles force required to achieve heel rise
	• Adduction and PF at TNJ to transfer load off of 1st MT head to the lateral column
	• ***INCREASES LEVER ARM OF PERONEUS LONGUS and WINDLASS MECHANISM to increase the tension to PF 1st ray to increase arch height***
	Complications:
	• Nonunion
	• Arthritis @ CCJ or STJ, can consider fusing CCJ
	   o could be due to improper graft size
	• Lateral column overload-strain greatest at lateral band of LPL
	      o 5th MT stress fracture
	• Sinus tarsi impingement 2/2 graft impingement
	• Overcorrection
	• FF varus —> increased lateral FF loading
	   o do not obtain full RF inversion at propulsion

Calcaneo-cuboid distraction arthrodesis (CCDA)	Pros: alternative to LCL to prevent CCJ arthritis Risks: nonunion, MT-cuboid arthritis, greater increase in lateral FF loading compared to LCL

Cuboid adduction osteotomy	
Kidner	see saggittal plane
Medial cuneiform closing wedge osteotomy	

Frontal plane	
Koutsogiannis (Kouts) aka Medial displacement calcaneal osteotomy (MDCO), aka medial calcaneal slide osteotomy (MCSO), aka Posterior calcaneal displacement osteotomy (PCDO)	**MOA:** • redirects vector of Achilles tendon from eversion to inversion • shifts WB surface medially (posterior aspect of the tripod) • support for PTTD • Greater effect on STJ, not MTJ • No sagittal plane correction **Indication:** reducible hindfoot valgus, without forefoot varus, stable MTJ **Technique:** • Perform in conjunction with FDL transfer, LCL, or gastroc lengthening • incision inferior to distal fibular tip, inferior to peroneal tendons, • Posterior fragment of calcaneus translated medially 1cm-1.2cm • 6.5 cannulated screw from inferolateral to superomedial (under hard sustentaculum tali) • tamp on lateral protrusion of proximal calcaneal fragment to prevent tissue/sural N irritation
Reverse Dwyer	medial closing wedge osteotomy
Double calcaneal osteotomy (DCO)	LCL + MCSO

JOINT FUSIONS:

TN fusion	**Strength:** Triplanar correction **Caution:** over-correction in adduction leads to poor outcomes
STJ, Lapidus, TN, NC, triple, pantalar	for more severe deformities
Miller procedure (NC and TMT)	corrects forefoot supinatus

Arthroeresis	**Definition:** • "limitation of joint movement", "internal orthosis", "internal orthotic device", "endorthotic" **Indications:** • children with PAINFUL flexible pes planus (collapsing pes planovalgus), REDUCIBLE RF valgus, TN sag, tarsal coalition • ONLY as adjunct, considering planal dominance (MCO + FDL transfer), heel cord lengthening • **Strength:** preserves joint function-does not negatively affect biomechanics of STJ, less morbidity, no risk nonunion, easy to perform, very stable • Useful supplement flatfoot recon in pts with systemic factors (obesity, DM, RA, smoking) **Contradindications:** • **angular deformity at knee**, torsional deformity, STJ arthritis, peroneal spasm, ligamentous laxity, MTJ instability, XS transverse plane deformity (TN uncovering) **Gait:** • talus PF and adducts (anterior displacement) • lateral process of talus hits the floor of sinus tarsi **MOA:** • Corrects excessive talar displacement, calcaneal eversion by preventing talus from rotating medially and plantarly, thus preventing lateral talar process from hitting sinus tarsi floor • restricts pronation while preserving supination • larger implant, greater decreased motion • Reversible, more common in children • protects medial ligaments **Technique:** • **Insert laterally in sinus tarsi just distal to posterior facet** **Complications:** • sinus tarsitus 2/2 to uncompensated FF varus (FF still tries to pronate), high implant removal rate (30-40%), hardware subsidence, loosening, foreign body reaction, cavovarus deformity **3 models:** **Self locking wedge**-any plug into lateral sinus tarsi to restrict STJ eversion by preventing contact of lateral process of talus with floor of sinus tarsi (Maxwell-Brancheau Arthroeresis (MBA), Gianni) **Axis altering**-angled peg to act as ramp to elevate floor of sinus tarsi, preventing talar PF, reducing calcaneal eversion. Bone resection required (STA-peg) **Impact-blocking**-limits anterior displacement of lateral talar process (Sgarlato mushroom)

Pediatric flatfoot, Congenital pes planus, calcaneovalgus
ET:
• MOST INFANTS ARE FLATFOOTED AND DEVELOP ARCH DURING 1ST DECADE
    ○ Self-corrects at 7-10 y.o due to increase in muscle strength, ossification of talus and navicular, decrease of ligament laxity
• **Internal rotation of hip**
• Tarsal coalition
• Congenital vertical talus (CVT)
• Accessory navicular
• Marfan's/Ehlers Danlos
CP:
• Avoidance of long distances, fatigue, medial arch pain, night cramps
• Heel in valgus
• DF'ed foot
• Gastroc tightening
TX:

Conservative:
- NSAIDs, stretching, kiddythotics, casting, AFO
- Plantarflexing foot to stretch out TA tendon
- Supra-malleolar ankle foot orthoses (SMAFO) for ankle valgus component

Surgical:
- Arthroeresis
    - o ONLY when pain (2-3%) in addition to evaluating planar dominance
    - o Ideal age: 8. Little lasting effect beyond age 10

Kidner foot, (accessory navicular, os tibiale externum, os naviculare secundarium, prehallux, gorilloid navicular)
The posterior tibialis inserts more __dorsomedially__ instead of plantarly, (creating more slack on the PT), weakening the PT supinatory power.

ET:
- Flexible flatfoot secondary to accessory bone at navicular tuberosity.
    - o Synchondrosis: connected by cartilage
    - o Synostosis: gorilloid navicular
- Trauma to PT area (athletics, obesity) can cause irritation
- pull of PTT on a synchondrosis can cause tension/shear

NH: Originally asymptomatic—cartilaginous precursor doesn't appear on radiograph until **9 to 11 years old**.

CP:
- Pain in shoes from rubbing navicular, acute injury
- Gorilloid navicular may skew talar covering measurement
- Can be confused with actual navicular fracture

Accessory navicular classification (Lawson[82])

Type 1	Os tibiale externum (in the PT tendon)
Type 2*	Synchondrosis (articulating ossification center) **2A:** PARALLEL attachment **2B:** PLANTAR attachment
Type 3*	Gorilloid navicular

*Types 2+3 = 70% of accessory naviculars

TX:
- Kidner procedure: (see PTTD) take out accessory navicular
    - o Debride navicular until flush with medial cuneiform
    - o Transpose TP more distal and plantarly, by rerouting through navicular or bone anchor
- Fuse the ossicle to the navicular: if asocial is large enough, using 1-2 fully threaded cannulated screws
- Trim off excess bone off navicular
    - o "faster" healing than Kidner because PTT not detached from insertion

Tarsal coalition, Peroneal spastic flatfoot
Tarsal coalition: bridge between two or more tarsal bones that restrict motion
Peroneal spastic flatfoot: major symptom of coalition, as PB tries to limit painful motion by immobilizing the STJ
Inflammatory condition at STJ/MTJ --> tarsal coalition --> peroneal mm attempt to splint STJ to reduce joint pressure --> peroneal spastic flatfoot

ET:
- Congenital
    - o Autosomal dominant mesenchymal failure to differentiate
    - o Accessory bones/ossicles incorporated into joint space
- Acquired
    - o Arthritis, infection, post-traumatic, neoplasm
- Tissue type
    - o Syndesmosis-fibrous union

---

[82] Lawson, J. P., et al. "The painful accessory navicular." Skeletal radiology 12.4 (1984): 250-262

- o <u>Synchrondrosis</u>-cartilaginous union
- o <u>Synostosis</u>-bony union, complete coalition
- <u>Extra or intra-articular</u>

EP: asymptomatic until the age of ossification due to flexibility found in cartilage

RF:

Associated conditions:
- <u>Symphalangism</u>-anklyosis of IPJs
- Carpal coalition
- Apert Syndrome
- Major limb anomaly

CP:
- Planovalgus foot type
- Tonic spasm of <u>peroneus brevis,</u>
  - o DX with common peroneal block to relieve spasm and pronated foot
- TRIAD (same as rigid pes pianus):
  - o 1) Pain (STJ, TNJ, sinus tarsi) 2) limited ROM (specifically inversion) 3) peroneal spasm
- Can be asymptomatic

PE:
- Hubscher maneuver: assess STJ ROM, ask patient to invert and evert feet while WB

DX:
- Radiograph (<u>Harris Beath</u>, lateral, obliques), confirm with CT, Tech 99
  - o Arthritic changes

Radiographs:

Coalition	Age	Radiographic Sign	Description
Talo-navicular	3-5	**TN beaking**-dorsal flag at TNJ	• mostly asymptomatic • second most common • Putter's sign
Calcaneo-navicular*	8-12	**"Anteater sign"**-lateral view **"Comma sign"**-MO view	Extra-articular "bar" Most symptomatic
Talo-calcaneal (STJ)*	12-16	sign" or "halo sign" continuation of talar dome and posteromedial talus with sustentaculum tali s of STJ clarity joint beaking eral talar blunting in lateral view (middle facet coalition) rris beath view: "angulated" (NON-parallel) medial and posterior facets CT is gold standard	MOST COMMON coalition (MIDDLE facet) pain at sinus tarsi broad, flattening of lateral talar process arrow posterior facet of STJ ball and socket ankle joint Harris beath XR view:
Calcaneo-cuboid			
Cubo-navicular			Extra-articular "bar"

*TC and CN each make up 45% of all coalitions

TX: SAME AS OSTEOARTHRITIS

Conservative
- shoe modification, padding, orthoses

Surgical
- Resection vs fusion: fusion if >50% of joint involved

<u>Resection</u>
- Better results:

95

- o   Age <14 with open growth plate, more prone to fail in skeletally mature
- o   Extra-articular "bar",
- Worse results:
  - o   Intra-articular coalitions, greater arthritic changes
- Grice Green procedure: extra articular STJ arthrodesis (EASTA)
  - o   indicated in age 3-14
  - o   fuses STJ without disturbing growth
- Badgley/Cowell procedure: for CN bar, excision of coalition with interposition of EDB

Arthroeresis

Fusion
- Better results:
  - o   Skeletally mature, intra-articular coalitions, greater arthritic changes
- Triple arthrodesis: 1) TN (MTJ) 2) TC (STJ) 3) CC (MTJ)
  - o   fusion of 2 joints: STJ + MTJ
  - o   Ollier's incision-lateral incision inferior to fibular malleolus over sinus tarsi to the base of 4th/5th MT. Good access to STJ and CCJ
  - o   6.5 or 7.0 cannulated screws
  - o   Fuse in VALGUS position to allow maximum medial column/first ray stability
  - o   TN joint is the key to motion of the triple joint complex (Astion et al, JBJS 1997[83])
    - ▪   most important/difficult to fuse (most common nonunion due to long re-vascularization time)
    - ▪   TNJ has the greatest ROM in the triple complex
    - ▪   Triple vs double: no need to fix CCJ
      - •   UNLESS FF abducted and CCJ distraction arthrodesis necessary

Astion (1997)	Degrees
normal TNJ ROM	37 degrees
% of STJ left after TN fusion	8%
degrees of ROM in remaining joints after TN fusion	2 deg
% of PTT remaining after TN fusion	25%

- o   Consider concomittant TAL
- o   Complications:
  - ▪   lose mobile adaptor, shock absorption
    - •   arthritis to ankle, knee, hip
  - ▪   pseudoarthrosis (CCJ)
  - ▪   AVN

Pes Cavus

Pes Cavus (Cavovarus foot), pes cavovarus
Neuromuscular imbalance leading to bony adaptation
- 60-70% neuromuscular
- Progressive vs non-progressive
- Spastic vs non-spastic
- anterior vs posterior

Anatomy:
- STRONG PTT/PL, WEAK PB/TA

---

[83] Astion, Donna J., et al. "Motion of the Hindfoot after Simulated Arthrodesis*." The Journal of Bone & Joint Surgery 79.2 (1997): 241-6

- PL is strongest deforming force, leading in PF'ed medial column

ET:

1) Congenital Neuromuscular disease (most common):
- CNS/LMN diseases:
- CMT (most common, progressive): damage to TA and PB. PL and PTT unopposed.
- Polio (non-progressive), myelomeningocele, muscular dystrophy (Duchenne), spinal cord disease, cerebral palsy, CVA, Friedrich's ataxia, talipes equinovarus, spina bifida, syphylis
- Spastic

2) Biomechanical (compensation for everted foot):
- Forefoot valgus, plantarflexed first ray, equinus, short limb length discrepancy, extensor substitution, flexor substitution
- loss of peroneus brevis leads to worst varus deformity
- Progressive

3) Acquired:
- Deep posterior compartment syndrome
- Tumors, brain/spinal cord disease, trauma, infection, iatrogenic
- Peroneals overpower TA/PT —> plantarflexed 1st ray —> "tripod effect"
- Spastic gastroc-soleus, TA/PT
- Stable

4) Idiopathic
- Approximately 1/3 of idiopathic cavus feet likely representative of underlying neurologic disorder[84]

NH: neuromuscular etiologies more progressive than biomechanics etiology

EP: 10% (Sachithanandam, 1995[85]) in general population

CP:

Japas Classification

Type of Cavus	Apex of deformity
Anterior cavus	Excessive PF of forefoot
Metatarsus cavus	TMT joint (Lisfranc), usually PF'ed 1st MT
Lesser tarsus cavus (MOST COMMON)	NC/lesser tarsals
Forefoot cavus	MTJ (Chopart)
Posterior cavus	Excessive DF of rearfoot (CIA >30), could be due to weak gastrocsoleus muscle
Combined anterior cavus	Multiple apices of deformity
Local anterior cavus	Portion of forefoot affected
Global anterior cavus	Entire forefoot affected

Coleman block test-with first ray hanging off a block medially:

Result of test	Implication	Hindfoot	Treatment
Heel varus corrected	Cavus 2/2 to FF valgus (PF 1st MT)	FLEXIBLE REARFOOT.	correct the forefoot

[84] Brewerton DA, Sandifer PH, Sweetnam DR. "Idiopathic" pes cavus: an investi- gation into its aetiology. Br Med J. 1963 Sep 14;2(5358):659-61.

[85] Burns, Joshua, et al. "Interventions for the prevention and treatment of pes cavus." The Cochrane Library (2007)

Result of test	Implication	Hindfoot	Treatment
Heel varus does not correct	Cavus 2/2 to RF varus	RIGID REARFOOT	correct forefoot and rearfoot

- 60% painful
- **Metatarsalgia**: forefoot pain, forefoot hyperkeratoses, sesamoiditis 2/2 PF 1st MT
- **Digital contracture** (extensor substitution via EDL)
- **Lateral ankle instability** 2/2 to ankle and STJ varus
  - o STJ, MTJ, and ankle OA
- Reverse Helbing's sign-lateral bowing of Achilles tendon
- Achilles tendonitis/retrocalcaneal bursitis
- Pseudoequinus
  - o RIGID cavus foot causes limited DF due to the RIGID plantarflexed nature of the FOREfoot (true equinus is measured from bisection of REARfoot to leg)
  - o The ankle has already "used up" the DF to compensate for the plantarflexed forefoot
  - o Not a true ankle joint limitation

DX:
- XR: increased Meary's/Hibb's angle, bullet hole sinus tarsi, increased CIA, posterior break in cyma line
  - o hindfoot alignment view
- Apex of deformity/center of rotation of angulation (CORA): look for "fault/breach" using the intersection of:
  - o Meary's lines (talus & 1st MT)
  - o Hibb's angle (calcaneus and 1st MT)

TX:
Ruch Classification

Classification	Location	Treatment
1. Digital Cavus	MT, MTPJ	digital fusion, MTPJ release, tenotomies, tendon transfer
2. Rigid cavus	Rigid PF 1st ray, RF varus	DFWO, Dwyer, STATT, peroneal stop
3. Severe global cavus	RF varus + FF valgus	osteotomy, triple arthrodesis, tendon transfer

Conservative
- RICE, AFO, steroid injections
- Orthotics: custom orthotics reduced foot pain and plantar pressure, increased foot function,

Surgical
- Soft tissue (Steindler stripping)
- Tendon transfer (Peroneal stop)
- RF osteotomy (Dwyer)
- Midfoot osteotomy (DFWO)
- Midfoot fusion
- RF fusion (triple, pantalar)

Soft tissue (flexible/semi-rigid cavus):

Procedure	Details
Steindler stripping	sectioning of plantar fascia, 1st layer of plantar muscles, LPL. First step of cavus foot correction SE: can activate Charcot
Subcutaneous fasciotomy	cute plantar fascia at insertion

Plantar medial release	release plantar musculature and ligaments at plantar medial foot
"Shapiro's Triple Procedure"	gastroc recession, plantar fasciotomy, PL release
TN capsulotomy	
Spring ligament capsulotomy	

Tendon transfers(flexible/semi-rigid cavus):

Tendon transfer	Details
Hibbs tenosuspension	EDL slips combined and transfered to lateral cuneiform EDB to EDL stumps + digital fusions (prevents extensor substitution HT formation)
Jones tenosuspension	• transfer of EHL to 1st MT head (distal EHL stump fused to EHB) + HIPJ fusion to prevent overpowering of EHL leading to hallux malleus) • EHL can also be transferred to TA, can also transfer FHL to proximal phalanx
Heyman tenosuspension	transfer EDL to MT necks
TATT	MOA: • TA to lat cuneiform • Decreases supinatory forces, increases pronation Technique: 3 incisions: 1. release from insertion 2. anterior leg to retrieve tendon 3. over lateral cuneiform for re-insertion SE: planovalgus if excessive transfer laterally
PTTT	• PTT through interosseus membrane to 3rd cuneiform (out of phase transfer) • PTT can also be transferred to TA
STATT	1/2 TATT to cuboid or peroneus tertius
Murphy	Achilles insertion to doral calcaneus just posterior ot STJ
PLTT	peroneus longus tendon inserted to base of 3rd MT
Peroneal stop, PL to PB transfer, peroneal anastamosis	PL tenodesis to PB. Decreases PF deforming force of 1st MT, increases eversion
FHL transfer	transfer distal phalanx to base of proximal phalanx
Gastroc recession/TAL	

Osteotomies

	Region of foot	Details

	Region of foot	Details
Jahss	Forefoot	CBWO through TMT
Japas	Midfoot	V osteotomy, apex at navicular, wings through cuneiform and cuboid. Slide distal piece downwards
Cole	Midfoot	dorsal CBWO through NC joint, cuboid
Duvries	MTJ	dorsal CBWO through MTJ preserves ROM of foot, sacrifices only NCJ, results in more normal ROM during walking
Dwyer	Rearfoot	lateral closing wedge osteotomy of calcaneus, for rigid deformity
Lateral column shortening	Lateral column	"Reverse Evans": remove bone from cuboid or calcaneus
DFWO	1st MT or all MT	For PF 1st MT (forefoot valgus) or all MT. Wedge extending from dorsal distal to plantar proximal. For flexible deformity
Scarf Z-shape calcaneal osteotomy		Combination of LCL AND MCSO Remove a 8-10mm piece, translate laterally 6-8mm

Arthrodesis:
- Hallux IPJ
- TN, CC, Triple arthrodesis + pantalar (longstanding deformity, with arthritis due to FF valgus compensation)

Ankle Pathology

Ankle sprain, Ankle joint capsule tear
*mostly sagittal plane ROM, but a good amount of transverse/frontal ROM due to lack of ROM at STJ (Lundgren et al[86])
ET:
- Low ankle sprain:
  - o   #1: ATFL (95%), #2: CFL/AITFL, #3: PTFL
    - CFL: DF + inversion, may also tear peroneal tendon sheath
    - ATFL: PF + inversion
  - o   Common in dancers due to peroneal mm weakness
- Medial ankle sprain:
  - o   Rare, associated with peroneal tendon pathology
- Talar anatomy
  - o   medial articulation-comma shape
- Tibia anatomy

---

[86] Lundgren, P., et al. "Invasive in vivo measurement of rear-, mid-and forefoot motion during walking." Gait & posture 28.1 (2008): 93-100.

- o   medial malleolus: anterior (larger) and posterior colliculus
- Ankle ligaments:
  - o   Deltoid (MCL):
    - **Superficial**-tibionavicular, tibiocalcaneal, superficial (posterior) tibiotalar.
    - **Deep**-deep anterior/posterior tibiotalar (strongest)
  - o   LCL:
    - PTFL, ATFL, CFL
- Joint capsule tear: due to hyper PF, such as when accidentally kicking the ground or trauma to anterior ankle with foot maximally plantar flexed

EP:
- Mostly found in elderly women, 2/3 are isolated malleolar

RF:
- Previous history of sprain
- High BMI
- Prevention: orthosis, peroneus brevis strengthening, proprioception exercise

CP:
- The more extensive ligament injury, the more difficult to WB, more swelling, more ecchymosis
- Sharp, shooting pain over ligament

Diaz Classification:

Grade	Ligaments
1	ATFL
2	CFL
3	ATFL + CFL
4	ATFL + CFL + PTFL

Grade	Anatomic	Findings	Treatment	Return to play
1	ATFL **stretch**		Functional treatment	2-4 weeks
2	ATFL+ CFL **partial tear**		""	6-8 weeks
3	ATFL, CFL, PTFL **complete tear**	+ ecchymosis - radiographic findings	""	8-12 weeks
Medial ankle	Deltoid ligament		Immobilization or walking cast/walking boot	6-8 weeks
High ankle	Syndesmosis	normal medial clear space	NWB CAM boot or cast x 2-3 weeks	4-8 weeks
High ankle	Syndesmosis	Wide medial clear space, tib/fib space	NWB cast 8 wks Screw removed @ 12 wks	Next season

Ankle sprain classification

Degree	Clinical Description
Mild	minimal functional loss, no limp, minimal/no swelling, point tenderness

Degree	Clinical Description
Moderate	functional loss, unable to toe rise, limp, swelling
Severe	diffuse tenderness, prefer to NWB

TX:

Ankle sprain functional treatment:

Treatment	Biology	Timing
RICE/NSAIDs	Minimizes inflammation for best condition for healing	Immediately
Brace in DF/neutral	Fibroblasts invade area to form collagen fibers	1-3 weeks
ROM exercise	Orients fibers, prevents the deleterious effects of immobilization on cartilage, bones, mm, tendon	3-6 weeks
Return to activity	Collagen maturation and remodeling	6-12 weeks
Prevent recurrence	Most dominant preventative intervention[87]	

Ankle fracture

DX:
- XR-medial clear space, talar position in mortise, tib-fib overlap
    - AP-ankle mortise and syndesmosis
    - mortise-fibular shortening,
- Bone san, CT, MRI

Physical exam	Finding
Anterior Drawer	>1cm OR >3mm compared to opposite side is abnormal
Talar tilt	>10 degrees OR >5 degrees compared to opposite side is abnormal
proximal squeeze test, proximal compression test	squeeze tibia against fibula at mid-calf, positive test is pain at distal tib fib **LEAST RELIABLE**
Distal compression test	compression at distal malleoli pain at syndesmotic ligaments
Eversion stress test, external rotation stress test	• Hip and knee flexed at 90 deg, stabilize leg, evert the foot against the fibula • pain at syndesmosis indicates injury • **BETTER (clinical) TEST FOR SYNDESMOSIS INJURY**

[87] Janssen KW, Hendriks MR, van Mechelen W, Verhagen E. The cost-effectiveness of measures to prevent recurrent ankle sprains: results of a 3-arm randomized con- trolled trial. Am J Sports Med. 2014 Apr 21;42(7):1534-41.

Cotton test, Hook test	• intra-operatively, clamp/bone hook to laterally pull on fibula to test integrity of syndesmostic complex by focusing on ANTEROLATERAL corner of joint
	• Also check for talar shift >3-4mm
	• **BEST TEST FOR SYNDESMOSIS INJURY**
Medial swelling/tenderness	• r/o deltoid injury
	• Medial tenderness DOES NOT predict deltoid rupture found in stress-view (DeAngelis)

Radiograph	Finding
Mortise	position foot in 15 degrees internal rotation
Medial Clear space, superior clear space (mortise)	>4mm is abnormal, both should be equal
Tib fib clear space (AP & mortise)	**Greater than or equal to 6mm** is abnormal **MOST RELIABLE**
Tib fib overlap (AP)	• **6mm-10mm 1 cm above ankle joint** or <42% fibular width is abnormal, indicates syndesmotic rupture • distance between tibial incisura and medial aspect of fibula • measure 1cm above ankle joint
Inversion stress view, Varus stress view AKA talar tilt (mortise)	>2mm, >5 degrees is abnormal = ATFL/CFL injury
Talocrural angle (lateral mall)	1) Angle between tips of malleoli and tibial plafond, normal is 8-15 deg 2) Angle between tips of malleoli and line perpendicular to tibial plafond: <83 is fibular shortening 3) within 2-3 deg of contralateral side
Shenton's line (fibular length)	Line continuous with **spur of lateral malleolus in ankle joint** with the tibial plafond
Dime sign AKA ball sign (fibular length)	Unbroken curve in the recess of the distal tip of fibula. Assesses fibular length and talocrural angle
Eversion/external rotation stress view, manual stress view (deltoid rupture)	**Indication**: • fibular fx, medial side tenderness but no medial mortise widening **Positive test:** • Look for: increased medial gutter space, decreased tib fib overlap **Use: deltoid rupture, syndesmosis injury** **CONS:** • false negative • Difficult to do (painful) in acute setting

Gravity stress view (deltoid rupture)	**Positive test:** • transection of superficial and deep deltoid >/= 2mm subluxation, 15 deg valgus **PROS:** • less pain, more effective. Lateral leg on pillow, allowing gravity to evert foot
WB stress (deltoid rupture)	**PROS:** • better at diagnosing "true" deltoid rupture • medial instability may be overestimated with gravity/manual stress views (false positives generated by partial deltoid rupture)
External rotation lateral view (posterior mall)	posterior malleolus
Double contour sign (posterior mall)	double contour of medial malleolus, indicates posterior malleolus fracture
CT scan	evaluate talus alignment with distal fibula
Tenogram	CFL rupture
Arthrogram	**Techinque:** • injection of dye into ankle joint, which should remain in joint. **USE:** • Only useful in acute ruptures while ligaments are still damaged, before fibrosis begins
Lamda sign	coronal MRI to diagnose latent syndesmotic ruptures >2mm of diastasis

CP:
- Swelling due to fracture: hematoma formation, not edema
  - Fracture blister
  - Ankle pinch test to check for swelling
- Check for peroneal tendon subluxation
- Poor prognosis
  - OCD injury of talus
  - injury of tibial plafond

Ottawa ankle rules:
Ankle XR needed if **pain at one or both malleoli PLUS:**

1) Age 55+
2) Unable to WB immediately after injury OR take 4 steps
3) Tenderness @medial/lateral malleolus, navicular, base of 5th MT

Danis Weber
- Above or below syndesmosis

Lauge Hansen*
- Cadaver study
- Forced movement of the foot in OKC with tibia stationary. Not accurate as most ankle injuries are with foot stationary and tibia moving against foot.
  - No reliable sequence of osseous and soft tissue injury predicted in SER mechanism[88]

---

[88] Kwon, John Y., et al. "A Cadaver Study Revisiting the Original Methodology of Lauge-Hansen and a Commentary on Modern Usage." The

- o Ankle fractures are produced by a combination of de- forming forces including rotation, angulation, axial loading, and translation
- Does not dictate treatment
- 10% of fractures cannot be classified using this system
- not perfect at predicting soft tissue injury

Lauge Hansen	Fx begins @	Danis Weber	Other
SAD		A	Most stable
SAD I	Lateral	A	TRANSVERSE fibula "avulsion" OR LCL rupture
SAD II	Medial	A	oblique tibia (no deltoid)
SER	(foot DF)	B	More stable
SER I	Anterior	B	Tillaux-Chaput/ Wagstaffe, AITFL
SER II	Lateral	B	spiral oblique fibula, (POSTERIOR spike seen on lateral), no LCL, due to lateral impingement of talus on fibula **MOST COMMON**
SER III	Posterior	B	Volkmann OR PITFL
SER IV	Medial	B	Transverse tibia OR deltoid rupture
PAB		B	
PAB I	Medial	B	Transverse tibia OR deltoid rupture
PAB II*	Anterior	B	Tillaux-Chaput/ Wagstaffe, AITFL ***OR PITFL**
PAB III	Lateral	B	oblique or COMMINUTED fibula, no LCL AP view-LATERAL spike, Lateral view-transverse fracture
PER	(foot PF)	C	
PER I	Medial	C	Transverse tibia OR deltoid rupture
PER II	Anterior	C	Tillaux-Chaput/ Wagstaffe, AITFL
PER III	Lateral	C	Maisonneuve fx, spiral fibula, syndesmotic rupture (PITFL tear), no LCL, due to tension on fibula
PER IV	Posterior	C	Volkmann OR PITFL

Ankle fracture terminology:
- DISPLACEMENT + ANGULATION

	Description
Tillaux-Chaput	Tibia from AITFL
Wagstaffe	Fibula from AITFL
Volkmann	Posterior tibia from PITFL

Journal of Bone & Joint Surgery 97.7 (2015): 604-609

Bosworth	Posterior fibula from PITFL, locked behind posterolateral ridge of tibia, preventing closed reduction of fx
Maisonneuve	Proximal fibula, PER III mechanism, complete rupture of syndesmotic complex is NOT necessary. Surgery NOT necessary
Pott's fracture/Dupuytren's fracture	Bimalleolar fracture
Cotton fracture	Trimalleolar fracture
Bimalleolar equivalent	rupture of deltoid ligament, more unstable than medial malleolar fracture
Coonrad-Bugg trap	interposition of PTT prevents reduction of medial malleolar fragment
Butterfly fragment	in PAB, triangular wedge of cortical bone part of comminuted fx. Created by two oblique fracture lines from a compressive bending force and a distracting force
Vassal phenomenon	Reduce primary fracture allows the other fractures to self reduce
Greenstick fracture	Incomplete fracture Only one cortex affected because other side is too soft to break Common pediatric fracture due to bending force
Torus fracture AKA "buckle" fracture	Incomplete fracture, "buckling" of the cortices Common pediatric fracture at the transitional zone between metaphysis and diaphysis
Stress fracture	Ill defined increased density
Minimally invasive percutaneous plate osteosynthesis for ankle fractures (MIPPO)	Decreases chance of wound dehiscence especially in DM patients or pts with poor vascular supply

TX:
Ankle fracture treatment s/p closed reduction

Time	Activity
4-6 weeks	NWB
6-8 weeks	Protected weight bearing
8-9 weeks	Full weight bearing in cast/boot
9-12 weeks	Remove cast

Closed reduction:
- Charnley technique: exaggerate, distract, reduce
- Reduce talus under tibia, align 2nd MT with tibial crest
- Prevent pressure necrosis of skin, prevent articular damage, reduce swelling
- If talus cannot be reduced —> SURGICAL EMERGENCY due to neurovascular/skin compromise
- Quigley maneuver[89]: in supine, externally rotated position, suspend entire limb on hallux which puts ankle through Supination, Adduction, Internal rotation

Sedation:
- IV Versed (midazolam) & morphine

[89] Bucholz, Robert W., et al. Rockwood and Green's Fractures in Adults: Rockwood, Green, and Wilkins' Fractures. Lippincott Williams & Wilkins, 2002.

- Hematoma block: 20 gauge needle at medial ankle joint medial to TAT, aspirate hematoma to confirm needle placement. Inject 12cc 1% lidocaine without epi. Just as good as conscious sedation
    - Nitrous oxide/general anesthesia
  - Knee bent
- Splint ankle in NEUTRAL position, avoid equinus
- ICE, foot pumps to minimize edema

Surgery:
- Perform surgery before swelling develops or after swelling resolves
  - best to wait for ~5 days post injury to allow soft tissue to recover from inflammatory phase
- Surgical indications
  - DISPLACEMENT:
    - Displacement (>2mm), angulation >15 degrees
  - INSTABILITY
    - Disruption of >2 parts of THE RING
    - Isolated displaced fibular fractures have good outcomes without surgery
      - XR overestimates degree of fibular displacement,
      - Deltoid holds talus in place
  - Shortened fibula (decreased talocrural angle)
  - Open fracture
SURGICAL GOALS
    - Fibular length (Yablon JBJS[90])
    - Ankle mortise (especially for high-energy injury)
      - 1mm lateral displacement of talus= 42% decrease in ankle articulation (Ramsey JBJS 1976[91])
      - 49% increase in joint contact pressure (Zindrick[92])
    - Lateral displacement of talus = increased medial contact
    - Syndesmosis

Pearls and Techniques for ankle fixation

Pearls	Technique

[90] Yablon, ISADORE G., F. G. Heller, and L. E. R. O. Y. Shouse. "The key role of the lateral malleolus in displaced fractures of the ankle." The Journal of Bone & Joint Surgery 59.2 (1977): 169-173.
[91] Ramsey, PAUL L., and W. I. L. L. I. A. M. HAMIITON. "Changes in tibiotalar area of contact caused by lateral talar shift." The Journal of Bone & Joint Surgery 58.3 (1976): 356-357.
[92] Zindrick, M. R., et al. "The effect of lateral talar shift upon the biomechanics of the ankle joint." Orthop Trans 9 (1985): 332-333.

	Pearls	Technique
Lateral malleolus	• TALUS FOLLOWS FIBULAR DISPLACEMENT (Yablon 1977) • fibula acts as buttress • Spiral oblique pattern makes interfrag screw effective • **Do not need to reduce if fx at midshaft or proximal fibula. <u>JUST REDUCE SYNDESMOSIS AND THOSE FRACTURES WILL SELF-REDUCE</u>!** • superficial peroneal exits crural fasica 12-14cm above ankle joint to split into intermediate and medial dorsal cutaneous N	• **QUALITY OF REDUCTION IS KEY TO SUCCESS** **Anterior approach**: avoid superficial peroneal N or AITFL **Lateral approach:** • Interfrag screws in lag technique perpendicular to fracture line • 1/3 tubular plate, 3.5 cortical screws to neutralize torsional rotational force • plate usually placed laterally • at least 2 bicortical screws proximally and 2 unicortical screws distally **Posterior approach:** • avoid sural N • **posterior plate aka anti-glide plate**-best stability, allows bicortical purchase. STRONGER than locking plates AND lateral plate • Risk peroneal irritation • unicortical screws distally to avoid entering lateral gutter **Lag screw only fixation:** • long oblique and non-comminuted fractures ONLY • for patients with good bone stock **Maisonneuve fracture:** • syndesmotic screw at distal fibula will reduce proximal fibular fracture **Tetracortical fixation (tibia-fib aka syndesmotic screws):** • 34% increase in energy before failure (Panchbhavi FAI 2009[93]) • good, cheap alternative to locking plate for osteoporosis, comminuted fracture **PAB and comminuted fibular fractures**: extra-periosteal, percutaneous fixation: **IM fibular nail:** • okay for non-comminuted fractures • technically difficult • promising for elderly, soft tissue compromise
Medial malleolus	• Bimalleolar equivalent fracture MORE unstable than true bimal fractures • up to 4-5mm clear space will do well with conservative treatment • 6-7mm clear space MUST ORIF	• Fixation (Ostrum et al[94]): 1) tension band 2) 2x 4.0mm cancellous partially threaded screws medial malleolar screw 3) K-wire • Anti-glide plate • Anteromedial approach: avoid saphenous V/N

[93] Stuart, Kyle, and Vinod K. Panchbhavi. "The fate of syndesmotic screws." Foot & ankle international 32.5 (2011): 519-525.
[94] Ostrum, Robert F., and Alan S. Litsky. "Tension band fixation of medial malleolus fractures." Journal of orthopaedic trauma 6.4 (1992): 464-468.

	Pearls	Technique
Posterior malleolus	**Anatomy:** • majority of fractures are triangular shaped involving the posterolateral tibial plafond (Haraguchi JBJS 2006[95]) **When to fix?** • fixate if >25% of articular surface (mixed opinions), reducing fibula may be enough • if fixated, need to fixate syndesmosis? • 70% stiffness restored with posterior mall fixation, 40% stiffness with syndesmosis screw[96] • >50% still had instability of syndesmosis after fixation of lateral, medial, posterior fragments (Meyer JFAS). Especially the case for smaller posterior mall fragments • <u>wise to assess syndesmosis for each posterior malleolar fractures</u> • double contour sign **How to measure fragment size?** • consider CT scan • externally rotated lateral view (Meyer JFAS)	**Posterior to anterior** • Better screw purchase than anterior to posterior • greater dissection • Posterolateral approach (between Achilles T and peroneal T): avoid sural N, lesser saph **Anterior to posterior** • Technically easier, (percutaneous clamps, cannulated screws) • Difficult to get all the threads in fragment without screw being too long/short
Deltoid ligament	• Deltoid complex is primary stabilizer of ankle (Michelson 2003) • **there is NO benefit to repair of deltoid ligament**	
Diabetics	**Most important factor**: NEUROPATHY • NOT at risk of complications unless >1 comorbidity (Jones) • 5-10% risk —> Charcot (Bibbo)	**Conservative**: TCC **Surgical**: • Better fixation-syndesmotic screw, locking plate • Prolonged NWB (6-12wks), then WB 2-3 mo in cast **Locking plate** • creates a "fixed angle device" • allows for unicortical screws to function as bicortical fixation and compression of plate to bone • NOT clinically superior to traditional plating
Pediatrics	possible epiphyseal fracture, short leg cast x 3 weeks	

• Post-op protocol
  o **Early ROM:**
    ▪ no clear benefit for earlier ROM vs immobilization x6wks
      • Pros: for younger patient, quicker return to work, better ROM, less DVT
      • Cons: increased wound complications
    ▪ No issues with protective WB <15 days[97]

---

[95] Haraguchi, Naoki, et al. "Pathoanatomy of posterior malleolar fractures of the ankle." The Journal of Bone & Joint Surgery 88.5 (2006): 1085-1092.
[96] Gardner MJ, et al., Clin Orthop Rel Res. 447:165-71, 2006.
[97] Starkweather, Michael P., David R. Collman, and John M. Schuberth. "Early protected weightbearing after open reduction internal fixation of

- Complications
  - Ankle malunion
    - <u>Overt</u>-talar shift
    - <u>Occult</u>-externally rotated distal fibula

Syndesmosis injury

LEVEL OF FIBULAR FRACTURE DOES NOT CORRELATE WITH LIKELIHOOD OF INJURY

ET:

- PER Weber C **or** SER Weber B
- **MOA**: EXTERNAL rotation + hyperDF (football, skiing)
  - stresses AITFL-pain with DF
  - degree of injury ranges from sprain—>frank diastasis
  - Mostly the AITFL (40%), also PITFL

CP:

- 10% of all ankle injuries
- frank instability or latent instability
- Isolated ligamentous injury OR associated ankle fracture
- 1-2mm normal elasticity with DF/PF
- Frequently mis/under diagnosed
  - can result in chronic ankle pain, arthritis

Anatomy:

- <u>Syndesmosis (5)[98]</u>:
  - Ligaments hold fibula within the tibial fibular recess.
  - AITFL (35%), PITFL (strongest, 42%), transverse tibiofibular ligament 33% (TTFL), interosseus ligament (IOL), interosseus membrane (IOM)
    - IOL-thickening of IOM, acts as spring which spreads the tib/fib during ankle DF. Shortest, but primary attachment between tib/fib
    - PITFL strongest, 42%:
      - Superficial (SPITFL 9%) + deep (aka TTFL transverse tibiofibular ligament 33%)

DX:

- Gold standard: intraoperative dynamic arthroscopic testing
- CT or MRI if rupture appears ambiguous on XR
  - 50-100% of 2-3mm diastasis not seen on XR, but on CT only

TX:

Goal: reduction of fibular in fibular incisura of tibia

Technique:

- Reduce with pelvic reduction forceps
- Underdrill only
- Insert screws parallel to joint as close to tibial plafond as possible, directed from posterolateral fibula to anteromedial tibia 25-30 degrees relative to coronal plane

<u>Syndesmotic injury + fracture:</u>

- Fixate when medial clear space widening s/p fixation of fibula
- Do not fix if bimalleolar fixation/deltoid intact (Yamaguchi 1994[99]) Enough soft tissue to hold syndesmosis together
- Over-tightening of the syndesmosis not possible (Tornetta 2001[100])
- NO NEED to fixate if posterior malleolus has been fixed

Boden criteria:

FIX	DON'T FIX

---

ankle fractures." The Journal of Foot and Ankle Surgery 51.5 (2012): 575-578

[98] Ogilvie-Harris, D. J., S. C. Reed, and T. P. Hedman. "Disruption of the ankle syndesmosis: biomechanical study of the ligamentous restraints." Arthroscopy: The Journal of Arthroscopic & Related Surgery 10.5 (1994): 558-560.

[99] Yamaguchi, Ken, et al. "Operative treatment of syndesmotic disruptions without use of a syndesmotic screw: a prospective clinical study." Foot & Ankle International 15.8 (1994): 407-414.

[100] Tornetta III, Paul, et al. "Overtightening of the ankle syndesmosis: is it really possible?." The Journal of Bone & Joint Surgery 83.4 (2001): 489-489.

FIX	DON'T FIX
>4.5cm proximal extension of fibular fx with deltoid injury	<4.5cm proximal extension with bimalleolar fixation
Only fractures proximal to 4.5cm need fixation due to longer lever arm resulting in greater instability	

Integrity of syndesmosis dependent on:
- Medial malleolar osteoligamentous complex (MMOLC)
- Posterior malleolus
- ***Do not need to fixate syndesmosis when either are fixated***

Syndesmotic screw (gold standard):
- **motion is necessary in the normal functioning syndesmosis
- **INDICATION**: No difference with or without screw (Kennedy[101], Yamaguchi[102])
- **MATERIAL**: No difference between titanium vs stainless steel (Beumer[103])
- **SIZE**: No difference 3.5 vs 4.5 (Thompson[104]).
    o 4.5 screw easier to remove, but greater irritation, less likely to real
- **NUMBER OF CORTICES**: no difference, (Beumer[105])
    o 1 screw across 4 cortices: higher chance of fracture, easier to remove
    o 2 screws across 3 cortices: better stability, better physiological movement
- **NUMBER OF SCREWS**: multiple screws for DM2, obesity, osteoporosis, Maisonneuve fracture, comminuted fracture
- **REMOVAL OF SCREWS**: No consensus, generally remove at 3-4 months
    o patients can complain of pain when screw left in
- **SE**: limitation of ankle ROM, broken screw, pain, screw removal, diastasis-loosening (sclerotic rim around screw on XR), heterotopic ossification, prolonged WB, synostosis, syndesmosis diastasis s/p screw removal, malreduction during screw insertion

Bioabsorbable PLA screw
- comparable to stainless steel
- $$$

Suture button devices:
- Zip tight or Tightrope (Arthrex)
- minimally invasive, flexible syndesmosis repair, no rates of malreduction
- earlier WB
- do not need removal of hardware
- Less malreduction of syndesmosis- 0% malreduction with tightrope vs 21% malreduction with syndesmotic screw[106]

Plate fixation

Isolated ligamentous injury (High ankle sprain):
- High ankle sprain: WBAT in boot/brace
- Latent/frank diastasis, good reduction: NWB 4-6 wks
- Irreducible: ORIF

Chronic syndesmosis injury
- syndesmosis widening >3 months s/p injury
- may be 2/2 to fibular nonunion
- continued stiffness, tenderness

[101] Kennedy, J. G., et al. "Evaluation of the syndesmotic screw in low Weber C ankle fractures." Journal of orthopaedic trauma 14.5 (2000): 359-366.
[102] Yamaguchi, Ken, et al. "Operative treatment of syndesmotic disruptions without use of a syndesmotic screw: a prospective clinical study." Foot & Ankle International 15.8 (1994): 407-414.
[103] Beumer, Annechien, et al. "Screw fixation of the syndesmosis: a cadaver model comparing stainless steel and titanium screws and three and four cortical fixation." Injury 36.1 (2005): 60-64.
[104] Thompson, Michael C., and Dirk S. Gesink. "Biomechanical comparison of syndesmosis fixation with 3.5-and 4.5-millimeter stainless steel screws." Foot & Ankle International 21.9 (2000): 736-741.
[105] Beumer, Annechien, et al. "Screw fixation of the syndesmosis: a cadaver model comparing stainless steel and titanium screws and three and four cortical fixation." Injury 36.1 (2005): 60-64.
[106] Naqvi GA1, Am J Sports Med. 2012 Dec;40(12):2828-35.

- syndesmotic calcification, adhesions
- confirm with CT

Pilon fracture, tibial plafond fracture
ET:
- AXIAL LOAD, driving talus into distal tibia
- severe soft tissue injury

Foot position	Tibial fragment
Dorsiflexed	anterior
Neutral	both
Plantarflexed	posterior

CP:

Look for injuries at calcaneus, tibial plateau, pelvis, acetabulum, spine

Varus deformity

DX:
- transverse slices CT (helps determine incision placement)

Ruedi and Allgower Classification

Type	Description
Type 1	No displacement
Type 2	Displacement
Type 3	Comminution, displacement, loss of tibial plafond

TX:
- <u>Fibular</u> reduction
- <u>Tibial plafond</u> reduction
- <u>Fill void</u> with cancellous bone
- <u>Stabilize medial tibia</u> (buttress plate)
  - Fracture line exits posteromedial-medial plate
  - Fracture line exist anterolateral-anterior plate

Ankle arthritis, ankle osteoarthritis, end stage ankle arthritis (ESAA)
ET:
- Post traumatic arthritis (70-80%), biomechanical, inflammatory/rheumatoid arthritis
  - Post traumatic-rotational ankle fracture with cartilaginous damage
- Ankle joint:
  - ankle surface area: 2 squared cm, 40% of articular surface of tibia.
  - contact area decrease with DF/PF
  - 3x body wt at heel strike, 5x at mid stance
  - ankle joint cartilage deforms 2/2 to WB to increase contact area
  - Ligaments that guide ankle ROM:
    - CFL, medial talocalcaneal ligament
  - Most important ligament during WB:
    - deep deltoid

EP:
- more common in younger patient
- much less common than arthritis of hip, knee

CP:
- coronal plane malalignment (varus deformity)
- lateral talar and fibular osteophyte
- ankle ligament imbalance 2/2 longstanding deformity

"Ideal" Candidate for TAR[107]

- Middle aged or older (sixth decade or older and , in general, the older the better)
- Low demands for physical and sports activities (e.g., hiking, swimming, biking, golfing)
- No significant comorbidities
- No smoking
- No obesity/overweight (normal or slightly increased body mass index; however, obesity is not a contraindication for this procedure)[17,26]
- Good bone stock with no risk factors for impaired bone quality
- Well-aligned and stable hindfoot
- Good soft tissue (e.g., no previous surgeries of foot/ankle)
- Well-preserved preoperative range of motion
- No neurovascular impairment of the lower extremity
- Reasonable expectations

Classification of TAR

- Surgical approach (anterior, medial, lateral, posterior)
- Bearing type (fixed, mobile bearing)
- Articulation resurfaced (superior, medial, lateral)
- External surface (hydroxyapatite, beaded, porous metal)
- Bearing surface (ceramic, ultra-high-molecular-weight polyethylene [UHMWPE], highly cross-linked UHMWPE)
- Sulcus type (none vs. normal vs. deep)
- Surface morphology (cylindric, conical, ellipsoid, spheroid)

TX:

	Methods	Strengths	Weaknesses
Total ankle replacement (TAR)	• Agility* • STAR (Scandinavian TAR)* • Mobility • Inbone 1&2* • Salto-Talaris* • Eclipse • Zimmer TM ankle* = FDA approved **Absolute contraindications:** previous ankle infection?, talar AVN, NM disorder (Charcot, Marfan, DM with neuropathy), ankle angular deformity >10 deg **Relative contraindications:** osteoporosis, smoking, DM, immunosuppression 2/2 steroids	-better ROM compared to arthrodesis -for young active patients -comparable results to arthrodesis -good for b/l ESAA, prev hindfoot fusion -conversion from AAD (difficult)	**Failure:** talar subsidence (posterior), loosening (worst pain), polyethylene wear Contraindicated in varus deformity >20 deg Hardware infection Higher re-operation (23%) revision, convert to fusion, BKA Loss of anterior tibial bone upon replacement Arthrodesis of syndesmosis Difficult to perform revision due to loss of bone stock
Ankle arthrodesis (AAD), ankle fusion	• Ankle fused at 90, 5 valgus • 0-10 ext rot • **post displacement** of talus to counteract pull of Achilles • Wedge resection of tibia to correct angular deformity • Charnley compressor • Trans-articular screws • Tibiotalar • IM rod/IM nail: (Wright medical Valor IM hind foot fusion nail system) • Calandruccio triangular compression device	-**Gold standard** -no difference in sports participation -6x more popular -better for pts with comorbidities	• Nonunion rate 15%-40% • STJ arthritis 2.8% (more compared to TAR) • 70% decreased sagittal plane motion • No clear consensus ankle arthrodesis leads to adjacent joint arthritis or alteration in gait[108]

---

[107] Coughlin, Michael J., Charles L. Saltzman, and Roger A. Mann. Mann's Surgery of the Foot and Ankle: Expert Consult-Online. Elsevier Health Sciences, 2013.
[108] Ling, Jeffrey S., et al. "Investigating the Relationship Between Ankle Arthrodesis and Adjacent-Joint Arthritis in the Hindfoot." The Journal of Bone & Joint Surgery 97.6 (2015): 513-519.

	Methods	Strengths	Weaknesses
Ankle distraction (diastasis)		-Symptomatic treatment	• 3 months in an external fixator • Poor long term results[109]
Blair procedure, Blair fusion	• Remove talar body • foot in 10-15 deg equinus • Tibial graft put into talar neck	-for talar body AVN, severely comminuted talar body fracture	
Supra-malleolar osteotomy			• Less predictable results, can risk hindfoot deformity
Allograft replacement			Inconsistent outcome, early failure

Talar subsidence grading system[110]

Grade	Findings	Treatment
1	no subsidence	Alter primary procedure (polyethylene thickness, revision of talar and/or tibial component)
2	subsidence not to the STJ	
3	subsidence at or inferior to STJ	STJ fusion

Osteochondral defects (OCD), osteochondritis dessicans, osteochondrosis dessicans, Osteochondral lesion of the talus (OLT)
"a lesion of talar cartilage and subchondral bone deprived of blood separates from the rest of the bone"
ET/RF:
• Traumatic (ankle injury):
  o **Compaction, shearing, avulsion**
• Nontraumatic
  o Microtrauma, endocrine deficiencies
NH:
        Damage —> uneven talar loading —> inc trauma —> more cartilage damage —> arthritis
        OCD decreases total ankle contact area and increases remaining contact pressure
        Size, location relevant for clinical outcome—central location worse outcome vs marginal
Extent of the depth of damage:
1. **Cartilage**: avascularity of cartilage, unable to heal but may remain viable from synovial fluid.
2. **Cartilage + subchondral bone**
   a. Injury immobilized: capillary penetrates bone fragment, healing occurs
   b. Motion at site of damage: displacement of cartilage and subchondral bone, formation of fibrous tissue, sequestering of fragment prevents capillary penetration, leads to AVN
DX:
• Hard to diagnose acute injuries (possibly no pain)
  o Diagnostic block into ankle joint

---

[109] Nguyen, Mai P., et al. "Intermediate-Term Follow-up After Ankle Distraction for Treatment of End-Stage Osteoarthritis." The Journal of Bone & Joint Surgery 97.7 (2015): 590-596.
[110] Gupta, Sanjeev, J. Kent Ellington, and Mark S. Myerson. "Management of specific complications after revision total ankle replacement." Seminars in Arthroplasty. Vol. 21. No. 4. WB Saunders, 2010.

- XR insufficient
- MRI needed to evaluate extent of osteonecrosis/AVN
- CT to evaluate damage to articular surface of cartilage of talus

CP:
- Ankle pain, giving away, ankle locking, stiffness, "catching"
- Persistent pain 8 weeks following ankle sprain

Berndt and Harty Classification

	Description	Treatment
1	Compression, overlying cartilage intact	Conservative
2	Partial detachment of cartilage	Conservative
3	Complete detachment of cartilage	Conservative/surgical
4	Displacement of fragment	Surgical

"DIAL A PIMP"	DIAL	PIMP
MOA	dorsiflexion inversion injury —> anterolateral lesion	plantarflexion inversion injury —> posteromedial lesion
fragment shape	SHALLOW, wafer shape	DEEP cup shape
stability	LESS stable, more likely to be displaced	MORE stable
pain	MORE pain	LESS pain
outcome	easier to treat	more difficult to treat

TX:
Conservative:
- RICE, NSAIDs, cast immobilization
Surgical:
- Smaller lesions: *Remove fracture debris and penetrate underlying bone*

Arthroscopy
Ports
- Anteromedial-medial to TAT, anterior to medial malleolus. Caution saphenous N/V
- Anterolateral-lateral to peroneus tertius, medial to lateral malleolus.
  - o Caution superficial peroneal N-intermediate dorsal cutaneous branch **(MC injured nerve in ankle arthroscopy)**
  - o PF 4th digit to visualize superficial peroneal nerve @ ankle near anterolateral port
- Anterocentral-between EHL and EDL tendon, avoid anterior tibial A and deep peroneal N

Instruments
- Cannula-rigid hollow tube
- Trochar-sharp tipped rod placed in cannula to pierce soft tissue
- Obturator-blunt tipped rod to penetrate joint. Protects capsule and prevents bending of scope
- Pistoning-moving scope in and out for orientation
- Sweeping-side to side movement to view anatomical areas
- Triangulation-brining scope and another instrument together through two different portals
- Irrigation-with normal saline or Ringer's (better for chondrocyte metabolism)
  - o Too much pressure can cause fluid to extravasate into peripheral tissue
  - o Egress port for fluid to leave
- Hemostasis-insufflation with epinephrine, radiofrequency ablation

Small lesions:
Excision and curettage
- Subchdondral drilling/microfracture
  - replaced with new FIBROcartilage, not hyaline cartilage
    - ▢ Fibrocartilage not as good as hyaline cartilage due to inability to resist compression. Poor long-term results
  - reserved for lesions with intact cartilage and underlying subchondral cyst
  - brings blood to lesion without cartilage disruption

Larger lesions:
Mosaicplasty aka Osteochondral Autograft Transplant System (OATS)
- a "cylinder" of hyaline cartilage from a NWB surface is transferred to the area of defect
  - restore mean contact pressure
  - several donor plugs can used to fill defect (4mm best, from ipsilateral talar donor)
  - knee can be used as donor site
  - 6-8 week NWB
  - Risk: for donor site morbidity

Talar en-block
- for recurrent OCD s/p OATS
- resection of talar wedge surrounding OCD and transfer a wedge from allograft

Lateral ankle instability, chronic lateral ankle instability, impingement syndrome
ET:
- Functional instability-symptoms of instability WITHOUT clinical/radiographic signs
- Mechanical instability-symptoms of instability WITH clinical/radiographic signs
  - **Scar tissue/fibrosis from previous ankle injury**
  - tendon injury (split peroneus brevis tendon)
  - nerve entrapment
  - synovitis
  - tear of perineal retinaculum
  - Hyperlaxity/strength deficits
- Ankle impingement
  - OCD
  - Soft tissue impingement-superior AITFL
- Risk—> arthritis if untreated
- possible STJ instability (check CFL)

EP: 20-30% of all ankle sprains
CP:
- Associated conditions: hind foot varus, perineal weakness, tarsal coalition, ankle arthritis
- lateral ankle pain
- feeling ankle is going to "give out"
- "clicking" upon eversion

DX:
XR (increased talar tilt), MRI
TX:

INSUFFICIENT EVIDENCE THAT SURGERY > CONSERVATIVE CARE FOR LATERAL ANKLE INJURIES

Conservative
- RICE, ice and NSAIDs better than either alone

Surgical
- Angle between ATFL and CFL: 104-132 deg
- Make sure to address concomitant deformities:
  - Varus heel—lateralizing calcaneal osteotomy
  - Tibial varum—tibial osteotomy
  - Forefoot driven cavus—address first ray declination (DFWO of 1st ray, Lapidus)

Anatomic repair	Anatomic reconstruction	Non-anatomic reconstruction

	Anatomic repair	Anatomic reconstruction	Non-anatomic reconstruction
Procedures:	-Brostrom -Brostrom Gould (Modified Brostrom)	-Use allografts (TA, PL, Achilles), or autograft (gracilis) to recreate original tendon	-Evans -Watson-Jones -Chrisman Snook
Indication	-Athletes -Non-severe injury -Restores normal anatomy	-When local tissues not enough for anatomic repair	-Mostly historical value only -Indicated when ligamentous destruction too much, for repair -Heavy demand -Prior repair -Inadequate tissue -Ligamentous laxity
Technique	**Brostrom:** ATFL repair: imbrication (overlapping) and suturing **Brostrom Gould (standard):** ATFL repair with inferior extensor retinaculum sutured to periosteum at distal fibula	-free tendon graft-autograft or allograft (semitendinosus, gracilis) -4.5-5mm diameter -tendon anchored at origins and insertions of ATFL and CFL	**Evans:** PB route through fibula ant->post **Watson-Jones** reroutes PB tendon through fibula (ATFL recon) **Chrisman Snook** reconstructs ATFL&CFL using split PB
Other	-long term stability (9yr) without impairment of ROM -Brostrom same postop clinical/radiographic outcomes as BG		-WJ and Evans do not replicate normal anatomy can —> stiffness -STJ/AJ arthritis -Increased ankle strength than simple repair -risk donor site morbidity and decreased PB strength

Peroneal subluxation, peroneal dislocation

ET:

- skiing (most common)
- Tendon can spontaneously re-locate

Eckert and Davis

Grade	Description
1	retinaculum separates from fibrocartilaginous ridge (most common)
2	fibrocartilaginous ridge detaches from fibula
3	avulsion fracture of fibula (least common)

Peroneal tendonitis, peroneal tendinitis

- Location of rupture and avascularity:
  - #1: Around fibula and calcaneus (**ENLARGED peroneal tubercle**)
  - #2: Around cuboid

ET/RF:

- OVERUSE: driving, ladder, motorcycle

- Varus foot-excessive STJ supination
- Chronic ankle sprain
- *Peroneus brevis is strongest everter of foot
- Ehler Danlos

CP: pain with eversion/abduction of foot

DX:
- MRI
- Oftentimes unable to fully diagnose until intra-operatively to assess tendon condition

TX:

Conservative: CAM boot, ankle brace WBAT, casting, steroid injection

Surgical:
- **Peroneal stop procedure** (PB to PL tenodesis)
- Tendon debridement
- **Peroneal tubularization**-tendon strengthened and wrapped with suture

Os peroneum syndrome, painful os peroneum syndrome (POPS)

ET:
1) os peroneum located within PL tendon
2) Fracture or diastasis of os peroneum
3) Tear/rupture of the peroneus longus tendon

CP: plantar lateral foot pain, partial/complete rupture of PL tendon

DX:
1) XR (os peroneum located at calcaneocuboid joint)
2) Ultrasound, MRI

TX:
- Casting
- Excision of os peroneum
  - Leaving the tendon in continuity
  - Tendon repair
  - PB to PL tenodesis

Achilles and Rearfoot Pathology

Plantar Fasciitis, plantar fasciosis, plantar fasciopathy, "heel spur syndrome" "painful heel syndrome" calcaneal enthesopathy

Anatomy:

3 bands:
- Medial,
- Central (5 bands, one for each metatarsal)
- Lateral (attaches to styloid process)

ET/RF:
- Activity-prolonged standing on feet
- Biomechanics
  - Equinus/heel cord tightness-fibers from Achilles' tendon continue to plantar fascia. Increased load on forefoot and windlass mechanism (Patel et al, FAI 2011[111])
  - Hamstring tightness-increased load on forefoot and windlass mechanism (Harty et al, FAI 2005[112])
  - Flatfoot/overpronation-rearfoot valgus/flexible forefoot varus
  - Cavus foot
  - Tibial varum
  - Limb length discrepancy
- Comorbidities
  - **Seronegative arthropathy (DISH)**- fat pad atrophy

---

[111] Patel, Amar, and Benedict DiGiovanni. "Association between plantar fasciitis and isolated contracture of the gastrocnemius." Foot & ankle international 32.1 (2011): 5-8.
[112] Harty, James, et al. "The role of hamstring tightness in plantar fasciitis." Foot & ankle international 26.12 (2005): 1089-1092.

- o   Obesity

EP:
- 15% of all foot complaints
- Female >> males

NH:
- Fibrofatty DEGENERATION, (not inflammation) of the plantar fascia origin with microtears and collagen necrosis
- Increased loads can also cause periosteal inflammation, fibrosis, heel spur
  - o   90% heal in 12 months

CP:
- **Poststatic dyskinesia-**"first step pain", pain in the morning, or at the end of the day
- Pain reproduced with windlass mechanism activation
- Deep achy pin-point pain upon palpation of plantar medial tubercle of calcaneus
- Plantar heel spur "enthesopathy" 75% located in FDB, above the plantar fascia
- mostly in MEDIAL band of plantar fascia
- RARELY bilateral
- R/O calcaneal stress fracture using squeeze test

TX:
Conservative (90% effective)
- RICE < NSAIDs < stretching < heel lift < (low dye strap) < OTC inserts < prescription orthotics < steroid injections < medrol dose pack < physical therapy < night splints < surgery
  - o   **Suppress:**
    - NSAIDs
    - Steroids-risk for fat pad atrophy, steroid flare, plantar fascia rupture (good!)
      - 3 injections per year
      - oral steroids (medrol dose pack)
    - Contrast soaks
  - o   **Stretching-**hamstring and calf _as well as_ plantar fascia stretch most effective
    - Plantar fascia stretch-belt or towel to forefoot, DF toes and massage plantar fascia
      - More effective than Achilles stretch (DiGiovanni et al, JBJS 2006[113])
    - Wall (calf) stretch-with knees straight, foot adducted, foot in inversion
    - Stair stretch
    - Rolling of (cold) can under foot
  - o   **Support**
    - Orthotics, supportive shoes
    - Goal is to reduce ground reactive force (GRF): deep heel cup, stiff medial arch, padded topcovers, heel cushion
    - Heel lift
    - Taping (good only for 24 minutes)
- ECSWT
  - o   Indicated when steroid injections fail
  - o   Alteration of small axons
  - o   Break down scar tissue, increase vascularity, leading to healing
  - o   RCT: not as good as steroid injections
- Radiofrequency coblation-localized fascia debridement
- Iontophoresis
- Platelet rich plasma (PRP)
  - o   stimulates chronic inflammatory phase—>acute healing

Surgical:
Plantar fasciotomy
SE: **lateral column pain (cuboid syndrome)**
1. **Endoscopic-**immediate WB
2. **Open**: plantar incision (In-step)—WB @ 3 wks
   a. perform with release of first branch of lateral plantar nerve (Baxter's nerve) release

[113] Digiovanni, Benedict F., et al. "Plantar fascia-specific stretching exercise improves outcomes in patients with chronic plantar fasciitis." The Journal of Bone & Joint Surgery 88.8 (2006): 1775-1781.

b. **Technique**: medial approach releasing flexor retinaculum over tibial N, abductor fascia over bifurcation of tibial N. Release 1/3-1/2 of medial band of plantar fascia. Also perform gastroc recession

Spur excision
Calcaneal decompression-relieves tension on the plantar fascia and TAL. 8-9 drill holes along lateral calcaneal body through medial cortex

Ankle Equinus, ankle equinovarus deformity ("horse-like" appearance of foot), spastic equinus
Passive ankle DF < 10 degrees
Anatomy:
- Gastroc/plantaris equinus-crosses 3 joints (knee, ankle, STJ)
  - Gastroc origin: medial/lateral femoral condyle
  - Plantaris origin: lateral femoral condyle
- Soleus equinus-crosses 2 joints (ankle, STJ)
  - origin: tibia, fibula

ET/RF:

	Spastic	Congenital	Acquired	Osseus	Soft tissue
Etiology	Cerebral palsy Duchenne	Normal first 3-6 months	**Diabetes**-non enzymatic glycation leading to Achilles tightening **Cavus foot**-psuedoequinus	Talotibial exostosis Talar neck exostosis	gastroc gastroc-soleus
Symptom		Toe-walking		hard and abrupt end ROM upon ankle DF with knee flexed and extended	

CP:

Equinus	Diagnosis (DiGiovanni JBJS 2002)
Gastrocnemius	< 5 deg ankle DF with foot in STJ neutral, knee extended but not flexed
Gastroc-soleus	<10 deg ankle DF with foot in STJ neutral, knee extended AND flexed

- Compensation through increased ROM at adjacent joints
  - Genu recurvatum
- **Steppage gait**-high knees for foot to clear ground
  - "Bouncy gait"-toe-walking, early heel off, short stride length
- ***Forefoot varus***
- Positive Meary's angle = FF equinus
- Lower back pain
- Compensation:
  - Pronation, flatfoot, bouncy gait, abducted gait
  - Lumbar lordosis, hip flexion, genu recurvatum

NH:
- Increased Achilles load —> decreased PL strength —> hypermobile 1st ray
- Inverts foot
- PF talus/navicular, DF 1st MT/cuneiform

DX:
- Silfverskiold test
  - maximally supinated RF

120

- o confirm while patient under general anesthesia
- Weightbearing lunge test
  - o Knee against wall sliding heel as far back as possible
  - o ~9-10cm from longest toe to wall

TX:

Conservative:
- Stretching, night splints, heel lifts, braces
- Serial casting-pediatrics up til adolescence
- Spastic equinus: botox injections

Surgery:

Treatment for Gastroc equinus

Strayer: TRANSVERSE incision, Suture proximal flap to soleus **CAUTION: NV bundle posterior to PT muscle: tibial N, posterior tib A**	**Silfverskiold**: RELEASE gastroc heads re-insert to proximal tibia	**Baumann**: recession of gastroc or soleus aponeurosis
McGlamery: (PROXIMAL) tongue in groove	**Baker**: (DISTAL) tongue in groove	**Vulpius**: V pointing proximally inverted V through gastroc aponeurosis

Treatment for Gastroc soleus equinus

Procedure (type of TAL)	Details
Hoke TAL	triple hemisection (medial, lateral, medial) 3cm apart from each other first incision 2cm proximal to Achilles insertion
Z plasty	in sagittal OR frontal plane
Hauser	section 2/3, medial 2/3 distally
Conrad and Frost	section medial 3/4 distally and lateral 3/4 proximally

SE: increased heel pressure —> ulceration

Treatment for spastic equinus

Procedure	Details
Murphy procedure	• Transfer Achilles insertion to dorsal calcaneus just posterior to STJ • Deep to FHL prevents tendon from recurrence of deformity • Decreases lever arm, good for spastic muscular forms of equinus (cerebral palsy) • Weakens triceps surae by 50%, MTPJ by 15% • SE: prominent posterior heel **Technique**: create a trough/groove over superior calcaneus just posterior to STJ for anchoring of tendon
Tendon transfers: TATT	tibialis anterior tendon transfer for flexible deformity, decreases supinatory force

Sinus tarsi syndrome, sinus tarsitis, sinus tarsalgia, lateral impingement pain
ET:

- Injury of <u>interosseus talocalcaneal ligament</u> inside the sinus tarsi
  - also injury of <u>cervical ligament</u> (anterior talocalcaneal ligament)
  - can also be chronic inflammation
- **<u>Status post inversion ankle sprain</u>**, joint instability causing repetitive strain, resulting in a pronated foot.
- Iatrogenic: arthroeresis implant

RF:
- planus foot type

CP:
- Subacute or chronic lateral ankle/STJ pain
- Pain with palpation of sinus tarsi, eversion of foot (close the STJ), not on inversion

TX:
- RICE
- Ankle stabilization-brace
- Orthotics with rear foot varus post to invert the foot
- Steroid injection into sinus tarsi
- surgical excision of contents of sinus tarsi (remove Hoke's tonsil)

STJ dislocation
Buckenham Classification

	Description	Frequency
Medial	"basketball foot", "acquired clubfoot", foot and calcaneus medial to talus	most common
Lateral	foot and calcaneus lateral to talus	second most common
Anterior and posterior	very rare	rare

Cuboid syndrome, cuboid impingement syndrome, cuboid peroneal syndrome, subluxed cuboid
ET: ankle sprain (cuboid forced plantar medial), excessive lateral stress 2/2 overuse, CAVUS, s/p medial band plantar fasciotomy
CP: tenderness along CCJ, calcaneocuboid ligament with concomitant perineal tendinitis

Haglund's deformity, pump bump, retrocalcaneal pain, retrocalcaneal bursitis
Painful bony prominence and bursitis of lateral posterior superior calcaneus above Achilles insertion
Haglund's deformity
- Triad: postero-superoLATERAL pump bump, AITC and bursitis

ET:
Haglunds:
- compensated RF varus
- compensated FF valgus
- rigid PF 1st ray

Retrocalcaneal pain:
- Retrocalcaneal bursitis-bursa between Achilles and superior 1/3 of posterior calcaneus
- Retrocalcaneal exostosis

XR: Positive diagnosis is positive parallel pitch + positive fowler phillip

	Fowler Philip angle	Parallel pitch line	Total angle of Ruch
Accuracy:	Less accurate	More accurate	
How to draw:	Line 1: ant tubercle to plantar tuberosity Line 2: tangent to Achilles insertion	PPL1: ant tubercle to plantar tuberosity PPL2: perpendicular to PPL1 with tip at superior most calcaneal tangent to talus	Fowler phillip + parallel pitch

Abnormal:	> 75 degrees*	When bone lies above PPL2	>90

TX:

Conservative:
- o Open back shoes, heel lift, orthotics, rocker sole shoes, NSAIDs, steroid injections, bursal aspiration, PT, topical anti-inflammatory

Surgical:
- o Extracorporeal shock wave therapy (ECSWT) with eccentric loading is best treatment if all conservative therapy else fails.
- o Achilles lengthening
- o Haglunds:
  - ▢ Remove inflamed bursa
  - ▢ Resection of bony prominence
  - ▢ Detach a portion of the Achilles
    - caution: "Chasing the bump" which can compromise insertion of Achilles
  - ▢ Keck and Kelly osteotomy

    - removal of sagittal wedge in calcaneus
    - Indication: structural cavus, high CIA
    - NWB for 3-4 weeks, BK cast 6-7 weeks
  - ▢ Duvries osteotomy-transverse resection of bump through MEDIAL or LATERAL incision
  - ▢ Fowler and Philip-transverse resection through POSTERIOR heel with Mercedes (inverted-Y) incision
  - ▢ Miller and Vogel-Keck and kelly with bumpectomy and ORIF

Tendon anatomy

- Achilles is body's strongest and thickest tendon
- Tendon rotates 90 degrees as it courses distally to insert on calcaneus. Soleus inserts medially to gastrocnemius
- Achilles does not have synovial sheath but instead a paratenon to allow for gliding activity
- Sural nerve crosses tendon 11cm proximal to insertion

Anatomy	Description
Paratenon	similar to tendon sheath, majority of BLOOD supply. preserve during surgery
Mesotenon	tissue connecting tendon to fibrous sheath
Epitenon	outer covering of tendon within sheath
Endotenon	tissue carrying blood vv surrounding small collagen bundles

Stages of Tendon healing (Tendon healing occurs in 4-6 weeks)

Stage	Pathophysiology	Physical therapy	Timing
1. Inflammatory	Neutrophil/macrophage infiltration, increased vascularity	Start passive ROM	1-7 days
2. Proliferative	Synthesis of type 3 collagen	Start returning back to activity.	1-2 weeks
3. Remodeling	Decrease in collagen, formation of fibrous tissue. Alignment of collagen fibers in direction of stress	HEALED	6-10 weeks

4. Maturation	Fibrous —> scar-like		10 weeks-1 year

Achilles tendinopathy, Achilles insertional tendocalcinosis (AITC) (tendinitis, tenosynovitis, insertional tendinitis/tendinosis, rupture, paratenonitis, enthesopathy)

*Achilles receives blood supply from muscle body proximally, calcaneal insertion distally, and from paratenon in between
Tendinopathy: includes tendinosis and tendinitis (histological findings).

- Tendinosis: micro tears in tendon 2/2 repetitive loading or stress on tendon. No active inflammation. MORE COMMON.
- Tendinitis: inflammation of tendon
- Paratenonitis: inflammation of paratenon (thickening), seen mostly in overuse injuries & athletes

ET/RF: MC: mechanical overload —> cumulative microtrauma
- Biomechanics:
  - o Cavus foot
  - o Hyperpronation
  - o EQUINUS
  - o Haglund's deformity/enlarged calcaneal tuberosity
- Lifestyle:
  - o Aging-decreased blood supply--#1 cause of noninsertional tendinopathy
  - o Male sex
  - o Improper footwear
  - o Athletic/work-related overuse: excessive physical training, training on unfamiliar surfaces, uphill walking/running (paratenonitis), high-intensity plyometrics
- Systemic conditions
  - o Seronegative arthropathy (insertional achilles tendinosis)
  - o DM, HTN, gout
  - o Obesity
- Chronic degeneration:
  - o Maximum load of tendon —> ischemia —> re-perfusion —> free radicals/oxidative stress—> inflammation (acute) —> degeneration/calcification (chronic)
- Ehler Danlos

CP:
- Concomitant bursitis, paratenonitis
- **Non insertional achilles tendinosis**: noticeable posterior bump, thickened Achilles tendon at watershed area
- **Insertional achilles tendinosis**: first step achy pain, pain worse going up a hill, shoe irritation

NH:
- Begins acutely as inflammatory process, then becomes chronic degeneration

DX:
- Radiograph: Spur formation at Achilles enthesis (insertional achilles tendinosis)

TX:
Conservative:
- Activity modification
- Medication: NSAIDs, oral steroids, topical anti-inflammatory
  - o NO EVIDENCE TO SUPPORT ANY TYPE OF STEROID INJECTION[114]
  - o Brisement-inject dilute anesthetic to break up adhesions[115]
- Orthotics:
  - o CAM walker/short leg cast-immobilize for 6-8 wks
  - o Heel lift-unloads Achilles T
  - o Open back shoes, orthotic devices, rocker sole shoes, night splint, posterior heel padding
- Tendon brisement
  - o Break up scar tissue to promote healing
- Stretching/physical therapy:
  - o Calf stretches could relieve tension on tendon
    - ▢ Eccentric-lengthening tendon while applying tension

[114] Maffulli N, Papalia R, D'Adamio S, Diaz Balzani L, Denaro V. Pharmacological interventions for the treatment of Achilles tendinopathy: a systematic review of randomized controlled trials. Br Med Bull. 2015 Mar;113(1):101-15. Epub 2015 Jan 12.
[115] Saltzman CL, Tearse DS. Achilles tendon injuries. J Am Acad Orthop Surg. 1998 Sep-Oct;6(5):316-25.

- ▢ Concentric-shortening tendon while applying tension
  - o Early active motion > dynamic splinting
- Other therapy:
  - o Extracorporeal shock wave therapy (ECSWT) with eccentric loading is best treatment if all conservative therapy else fails
  - o PRP injections (low evidence)
  - o Radiofrequency coblation

Surgical*:
- Reserve only for chronic cases
- LONG RECOVERY (need to detach and re-attach Achilles)
- *Key is to preserve paratenon, and caution not to damage skin over tendon

Procedures:
- **Tendoscopy**-excision of inflamed paratenon, release of plantaris tendon
- Release of adhesions
- Debridement of pathologic tissue and debulking of nodularity (non-insertional achilles tendinosis). Up to 50% of tendon can be debrided without risk of rupture
- Exostectomy-remove the AITC spur (2 yr recovery rate)
- Remove retrocalcaneal bursa
- FHL tendon transfer
  - o Low muscle belly of FHL increases tendon vascularity

Calcaneal bursitis, retrocalcaneal bursitis, subcutaneous calcaneal bursa

Type	Location
Retrocalcaneal bursitis	Subtendinous, between calcaneus and Achilles tendon
Subcutaneous bursa	in the subcutaneous layer between Achilles tendon and skin

ET: trauma, poor fitting shoes, arthritis, sports
DX: **"two finger squeeze test"**-apply medial and lateral pressure anterior to Achilles tendon
TX: RICE, NSAIDs, pads, steroid injection, heel lift
Surgical:
- Decompression of bursa
- Similar procedures for AITC

Achilles' tendon rupture, Achilles rupture, Chronic Achilles tendon rupture, Delayed Achilles tendon rupture
Rupture: occurs 2-6 cm proximal to insertion @ calcaneus, the "watershed area"
- Most common etiology: degenerative tendinopathy
- Acceleration—>deceleration mechanism in sports
- 99% of time, plantaris is spared because it is more anterior, creating a shorter lever arm

Chronic: untreated rupture >4 weeks
- Due to lack of pain, 25% ruptures go undiagnosed due to lack of pain
- Excessive scar tissue
- Surgical indication
- Decreased PF strength

ET/RF:
- Same as those causing AITC
- TRAUMA
  - o Landing on a PF foot
  - o Excessive PF with the foot planted
  - o Abrupt DF
- Systemic:
  - o HLD (xanthoma), gout, RA, hyperTH, CKD
- Medication:
  - o Steroids, fluoroquinolone (inhibit tenocyte metabolism)
- PMHx: men, elderly

EP: Middle aged athletic men (Weekend Warrior)
CP: feeling like got kicked in the back of the foot

EXAM:
- Mattle's test-pt prone, knee bent. XS DF = positive test
- Simmond's test-pt prone, XS DF = positive test
- Thompson squeeze test-pt in prone, knee bent, squeeze calf. Caution false test if accessory muscles are squeezed
  - POSITIVE: rupture, lack of DF
  - NEGATIVE: normal test, DF
- Brien needle test-place needle in gastroc-soleus, above the perceived rupture site
- Palpable dell-caution false negative if hematoma present
- "Hatchet strike" defect
- Unable to PF

DX
- MRI
- Radiograph:
  - **Toygar's angle:** based off of posterior skin of the ankle: <150 deg
  - **Arner's sign:** insertion of achilles curves away from posterosuperior calcaneus
  - Kager's triangle-borders of triangle (Achilles, superior calcaneus, FHL) will be ill-defined.

Kuwada Classification

	Description	Treatment
1	Partial tear, MOST COMMON (50%)	NWB cast PF 15 degrees
2	Complete tear <3 cm	Krackow, Bunnel, Kessler stitch
3	Tear 3-6 cm	Autograft (plantaris), graft jacket
4	Tear >6 cm	V-Y gastroc recession, Strayer
	Chronic rupture >4 weeks	FHL transfer, V-Y

TX:
Conservative (~18% re-rupture):
  - for inactive, elderly
  - Early WB and early ROM to prevent adhesions and tendon atrophy
    - However, tx during swelling could —> rupture. Wait for inflammation to resolve
  - **Willits protocol, JBJS 2010**[116]: accelerated functional rehab and nonoperative treatment just as effective as surgical
  - **If functional rehab with early ROM employed,** rerupture rates are equal for surgical and non-surgical patients[117]

Surgical (~2% re-rupture):
  - **Open repair less rerupture rates (3.6%) than nonoperative treatment (8.8%)**[118]
  - Better functional outcomes than non-surgical
  - For chronic tears
  - For active, younger patient
  - Technique:
    - Incision medial to Achilles tendon: avoid sural N, lesser saphenous vein, prevent adhesions, wound dehiscence
    - Dissect through epitenon

Tendon appearance	Chronicity of injury
mop-end	acute (days)
organized	1 week
chronic	necrotic

Surgical vs nonsurgical treatment[119]

[116] Willits, Kevin, et al. "Operative versus nonoperative treatment of acute Achilles tendon ruptures." The Journal of Bone & Joint Surgery 92.17 (2010): 2767-2775.
[117] Soroceanu A, et al. J Bone Joint Surg Am. 2012 Dec 5;94(23):2136-43.
[118] Wilkins R, Bisson LJ. Am J Sports Med. 2012 Sep;40(9):2154-60.

	Operative Treatment	Nonoperative Treatment
TABLE II Comparison of Operative and Nonoperative Treatment of Acute Achilles Rupture*		
Advantages	Improved functional outcome (e.g., return to sport). Faster return to work. Decreased rerupture rate (depending on protocol)	No complications related to surgery. Lack of scar
Disadvantages	Invasive (major and minor complications of surgery, especially wound-related). Greater cost	Greater likelihood of patient dissatisfaction. Adherence to functional rehabilitation protocol necessary for good outcome

*The choice between operative and nonoperative management of acute Achilles tendon rupture remains controversial, with certain advantages and disadvantages ascribed to each modality.

Technique	Details
Krackow	Strongest. Suture fails at rupture site giftbox suture (modified Krackow): suture knot tied AWAY from rupture site
Bunnell	criss-cross stitch to prevent shearing of suture through tendon
Kessler	

Adjunctive procedures (for delayed Achilles rupture)

Procedure	Details
V-Y gastroc lengthening	Especially useful for gaps 3-5cm
Silfverskoid	1 strip of gastroc aponeurosis
Lindholm	multiple strips of gastroc aponeurosis
Bugg and boyd	fascia lata strips join ruptured tendon
Bosworth	strip of gastric tendon freed proixmally flapped distally
FHL transfer	Most common procedure + gastroc lengthening stronger than FDL, lower muscle belly = better vascularity
PB transfer	
Graft jacket	For large gaps >10cm, allograft augmentation
Pegasus	equine pericardium
Lynn	Plantaris agumentation

- ****Postoperative care:**
  - Anterior short leg splint
  - Early ROM in brace:
    - Decreases adhesions and makes tendons stronger

---

[119] Uquillas, Carlos A., et al. "Everything Achilles: Knowledge Update and Current Concepts in Management." J Bone Joint Surg Am 97.14 (2015): 1187-1195.

- Increases collagen fibers
- Orients collagen fibers parallel to tendon's longitudinal axis
- Inhibits adhesions around tendon
- Increase tendon strength
- Increase tendon vascularity
  o DO NOT immobilize in cast
  o results in shorter rehab time
- Most common surgical complication:
  o Wound dehiscence due to poor soft tissue envelope between tendon and dermis
  o High risk DVT

Polymyalgia rheumatica
EP: 50+ y.o.
CP: aching, morning stiffness > 1 hour in shoulders/pelvic girdles/neck, fever, fatigue, weight loss for at least 1 month
   Often occurs concurrently with giant cell arteritis (vision loss, stroke, aneurysm)
DX: elevated ESR/CRP
TX: glucocorticoids—prednisone and prednisolone

Trauma

Metatarsal fracture
TX:
- Close reduce to correct sagittal and transverse displacement
- If unable to reduce, ORIF with pinning

5th Metatarsal
Jones fracture
ET:
- Large ground reactive force with failure of stationary foot to evert
- Torsion at the 5th MT as a stabilizer of the foot
- Difficulty healing:
  o Watershed area of intraosseus blood supply to the metaphyseal region
  o mechanical pulling of PB
  o Intraosseus circulation: 1) periosteal plexus, 2) nutrient artery, 3) metaphyseal/epiphyseal arteries
RISK: MT adductus foot type, cavovarus foot, genu varum, hind foot varus
CP: Transverse, extra-articular fracture 1.5cm distal to 5th MT tuberosity at the metaphyseal-diaphyseal junction
TX:
- Conservative: NWB cast for 6-8 weeks
  o NWB to prevent PB from pulling on bone (DeVries et al, JFAS 2015[120])
    ▪ reserved only for acute Jones
    ▪ many of these may —> nonunion
    ▪ plantar lateral cortex last to heal
- Surgical (>2mm displacement)
  o IM screw—4.5 cancellous is narrowest that should be selected (Scott et al, JFAS 2014[121])
    ▪ increasing diameter does NOT increase pull-out strength
  o External fixation
  o *a component of MAA makes fixation easier)
  o **Trephine arthrodesis** with graft from calcaneus[122]
    ▪ remove a cylinder of bone from both sides of fracture, fill with cancellous autograft from calcaneus

[120] DeVries, J. George, et al. "The Fifth Metatarsal Base: Anatomic Evaluation Regarding Fracture Mechanism and Treatment Algorithms." The Journal of Foot and Ankle Surgery 54.1 (2015): 94-98
[121] Scott, Ryan T., Christopher F. Hyer, and Shyler L. DeMill. "Screw Fixation Diameter for Fifth Metatarsal Jones Fracture: A Cadaveric Study." The Journal of Foot and Ankle Surgery (2015)
[122] http://www.podiatrytoday.com/rethinking-our-approach-jones-fractures-facilitate-shorter-post-op-recovery

Stewart Classification (5th MT fractures)

	Location	Description	Mechanism
1	E (extra-articular)	Jones fracture **Risk:** arthritis if enters 4th/5th MT space	ground reactive force with failure of foot to evert
2	I (intra-articular)	Intra-articular fracture of 5th MT base	shearing force with PB contracture
3	E	Avulsion fx of styloid process MOST COMMON of 5th MT fx (90%)	LATERAL BAND OF PLANTAR FASCIA reflex contracture of PB
4	I	Intra-articular comminuted fracture	crush injury
5	O	Apophysis injury in children	

Torg Classification (5th MT diaphyseal stress fracture)

	Description	XR
Type 1	acute injury	narrow fracture line
Type 2	delayed union (6mo)	widened fracture with IM sclerosis
Type 3	non-union (9 mo)	sclerotic obliteration of IM canal

Lawrence and Bott (location)

	Description	Mechanism	Treatment
Type 1	avulsion	LATERAL BAND OF PLANTAR FASCIA reflex contracture of PB	walking as tolerated in walking cast or CAM boot, pain as guide (Kaiser Vallejo)
Type 2	Jones	ground reactive force with failure of foot to evert	walking as tolerated in walking cast
Type 3	diaphysis	chronic stress, repetitive distractive forces	

Avulsion fracture, Dancer's fracture, pseudo-Jones fracture

ET:
- Due to pulling of lateral band of plantar fascia
- Inversion injury when foot attempts to stabilize foot creating a push-pull mechanism
- Blood supply: 4th plantar MTA, mostly @ plantarmedial diaphysis

CP:
- MC 5th MT fracture (90%)

TX:

Conservative:
- Immobilization, WBAT (DeVries et al, JFAS 2015[123])
- Walking boot better than short leg cast

---

[123] [123] DeVries, J. George, et al. "The Fifth Metatarsal Base: Anatomic Evaluation Regarding Fracture Mechanism and Treatment Algorithms." The Journal of Foot and Ankle Surgery 54.1 (2015): 94-98

Surgical:
- Tension band
  - Locking compression distal ulnar hook plate (Lee et al, JFAS 2014[124])

Tailor's Bunion, bunionette

ET:
- Genetics
  - Structural (Fallat classification)
  - Prominent lateral condyle of 5th MT head, lateral bowing of 5th MT, splay foot deformity (increased IM angle), PF 5th MT
  - Biomechanical: varus 5th toe, HAV leading to pronated 5th MT, hindfoot varus, flatfoot

Fallat classification

	Description	Frequency
1	Enlarged 5th MT head	27%
2	Lateral bowing	23%
3	Increased IM angle	50%
4	Combined	

DX:
- ▢ Lateral deviation angle (LDA): 2.64 normal, 8 abnormal
- ▢ 5th MT IMA: 7 is normal

Angle	Abnormal	Normal
Lateral deviation angle (LDA) (5th MT head & medial cortex)	>8	3
Fallat and Buckholz angle (4th MT and medial cortex of 5th)	8.05	<7 (2.64)
5th MT IMA	8.71	<7 (6.47)

CP:
- No pain or pain exacerbated by footwear, swelling, callus formation
- Tenderness on palpation of lateral 5th MT head, overlying adventitial bursa, plantar hyperkeratotic lesion, adductovarus

TX: shoegear change, padding, callus debridement, orthoeses, injection into bursa, NSAIDs

Surgical:

Procedure	Description
Exostectomy	remove lateral eminence
Arthroplasty	remove part/whole 5th MT head
Davis	reverse silver
Dickson and Dively	Davis + removal of bursa
DeVries	removal of lateral plantar condyle
Amberry	Davis + removal of base of proximal phalanx

---

[124] Lee SK, Park JS, Choy WS. Locking compression plate distal ulna hook plate as alternative fixation for fifth metatarsal base fracture. J Foot Ankle Surg 53:522–528, 2014.

Procedure	Description
McKeever	resection of 1/2-2/3 of 5th MT
Reverse Hohmann	transverse osteotomy in neck
Reverse Wilson	
Reverse Austin	
Long oblique distal osteotomy (LODO)	Weil osteotomy-like cut at the MT neck

Lisfranc fracture, lisfranc injury, lisfranc dislocation, lisfranc subluxation
Wide spectrum of injuries (sprain, dislocation, bony avulsion)
Anatomy:
- Lisfranc complex composed of dorsal (weakest), plantar (strongest), and interosseus (strongest) ligaments
    - Plantar lisfranc ligament strongest interosseus TMT ligament
    - The 2nd TMT joint is the **keystone of the arch**, wedged between medial/lateral cuneiforms. There is NO interosseus ligament between 1st and 2nd MT

ET:
- Most injuries are in DORSAL direction
- Forced abduction
- Twisting + axial loading of a PF foot
- Eversion/pronation (indirect trauma)
- Motor vehicle accident (direct, high trauma)

CP:
- "Plantar ecchymosis sign" (delayed)
- "Apprehension sign" with FF DF and abduction
- Stress exam of mid foot —> unstable TMT joint with pronation/eversion
- Ligamentous injury easily diagnosed as "foot sprain"
- MEDICAL EMERGENCY: R/O compartment syndrome

NH:
- #1 complication: ARTHRITIS 2/2 to flat-on-flat design of cuneiforms
    - Missed in 20% of cases leading to poorer function
    - planovalgus deformity, forefoot abduction

DX:
Radiograph:
- AP, lateral, medial oblique, pronation-abduction (FF abduction) stress view
    - Compare with opposite side
- AP view:
    - 1st MT and medial cuneiform aligned medially and laterally
        - 2nd MT and medial border of middle cuneiform
        - Space between 1st and 2nd MT should be equal to space between medial and intermediate cuneiform
- Medial oblique view:
    - 4th MT and medial border of cuneiform in medial oblique view
        - lateral border of 3rd and lateral border of lateral cuneiform
        - Lateral view:
            - TMTJ should be linear
- "Fleck sign"—fleck avulsion from base 2nd MT
- >2mm gap between 1st and 2nd MT is significant, needs surgery
- Dorsal step off of 2nd MT

CT scan:
- ANYTIME there is fracture at MT base, questionable extent of involvement at TMTJ
- for peri-operative planning

Hardcastle/Quenu and Kuss classification

	Hardcastle	Quenu and Kuss	Description of injury
A	Total	Homolateral	Disruption of entire TMJ (usually lateral) MOST COMMON
B	Partial	Isolated	B1: Medial displacement of 1st MT B2: lateral displacement MT 2-4
C	Divergent	Divergent	C1: (partial)1st MT medial, 2nd MT lateral C2: (total) 1st MT medial, ALL lesser MT lateral

TX:
For severe injuries, consider initial percutaneous pinning while waiting for surgery to prevent further displacement 2/2 swelling
Conservative (uni-directional instability, <2mm displacement):
- put in Jones' compression dressing
- conservative tx risk arthritis

Surgical (plantar instability, >2mm displacement):
- 3 incisions: medial to 1st, 2nd interspace, 4th interspace
- ORIF (better clinical outcome than conservative tx)
  - Earlier return to work
  o However, more re-operative rates, osteoarthritis rates, and conversion to arthrodesis (Henning)
- Primary arthrodesis of 1st-3rd TMT joints > ORIF (Coetzee)
  a. Contraindication: uni-directional instability
- Fuse only 1-3 because of their immobility
- DO NOT fuse 4-5 because they are more "essential" (mobile)
  - Increased stiffness of midfoot
  - K-wires and screws can be removed @ 8 wks s/p

Pantalar dislocation
- Complete dislocation of talus at ankle, STJ, and TNJ without concomitant talar fracture

Talar fracture

	Neck	Head	Body	Lateral process	Posterior process
ET	Axial load + hyperdorsiflexion "AVIATOR'S ASTRALAGUS"	1) crush (compression) 2) axial load on navicular (shear)	1) osteochondral 2) comminuted	see sneppen classification	shepard's/cedell fracture, forced PF of foot
EP	most common (50%), similar rates of arthritis and AVN as body fx		Similar rates of arthritis and AVN as neck fx		Sneppen 3
CP/TX	Canale XR view		NWB short leg cast 6-10 weeks		pain with DF big toe, WBAT 4-6 wks

Part of talus	Blood supply
Head/neck	**DP, ATA**
Body	A of tarsal canal (branch of **PTA**) A of sinus tarsi (branch of **peroneal A**),

Posterior	Peroneal A, calcaneal branches of PTA

DX:
Canale view: AP view with foot PF, pronated 15 degrees, to view angular deformity of talar neck

NH:
- o High rate of open fractures (up to 50% of cases)
- o Rule out compression of tarsal tunnel
- o Complications:
  - #1: Ankle/STJ arthritis
  - AVN (takes 6-8 weeks to appear in radiographs)
    - **Hawkin's sign**-subchondral sclerosis on AP view @ 6-8 wks indicates healing. Okay to r/o talar AVN
    - No relationship between timing of surgery and risk of AVN
  - Osteonecrosis

TX:
- SURGICAL EMERGENCY—2/2 protrusion of bone against skin causing skin necrosis, PROMPT REDUCTION OF FRACTURE
- Consider titanium screws so that MRI can be used to evaluate for AVN

Talar neck fracture

Hawkin's classification (talar neck)

Type	Displacement	Treatment	Risk for AVN*
I	No displacement	6-8wks NWB cast	12% (1 vv disrupted)
II	Displacement of STJ, or ANY displacement (medial more common)	Close reduce, percutaneous screws 6-8wks NWB cast. ORIF most likely needed 3.5mm screws posterior→anterior provides better fixation Anterior→posterior avoids vv, visualizes fracture. LAG SCREW	42% (2 vv disrupted)
III	STJ and ankle joint (talar body posterior medially) (>50% open fracture)	Surgery Consider medial malleolar chevron osteotomy	91% (3 vv disrupted)
IV	STJ, ankle, and TN joint (Canale & Kelly)	Surgery Pin TNJ	91% (vv to body, head, neck disrupted)

*risk of AVN increases in stepwise fashion
Lateral vs medial approach:

Talar body fracture
Sneppen Classification (talar body)

Group	Description	Mechanism	TX
I	OCD talar dome	COMPRESSION	
II	Body (coronal/sagittal)	SHEAR, severe DF	
III	Posterior tubercle (Shepard or Cedell)	severe PF Shepard-posterolateral Cedell-posteromedial	

IV	Lateral process	Snowboarder's fracture DF and eversion misdiagnosed as ankle sprain	NWB, ORIF, or excision
V	Crush		

Talar posterior process fracture, Shepard fracture, Steida's process fracture

Fracture of the posterior lateral talar process by the FHL

ET:
- R/O os trigonum
  1) Forced plantar flexion with compression of talar posterior process between the posterior malleoli and calcaneal tuber
  2) Forced DF leads to avulsion via PTFL

CP: pain with hallux DF

Nutcracker sign-pain with forced ankle PF

Navicular fracture

Anatomy: plantar-central 1/3 navicular is avascular

ET: abnormal spring ligament function, abnormal PTT, excess pronation.

MOA: excess force on 2nd MT—>middle cuneiform—>middle navicular—>navicular stress fracture

EP: Male athlete

CP: confused with type II accessory navicular (synchondrosis)

Nutcracker fracture: of cuboid and calcaneal anterior process

Watson and Jones classification of navicular fracture

Watson Jones	Description	MOA	Image
Type 1	Tuberosity	eversion 2/2 PTT	
Type 2	Dorsal lip avulsion fracture	frontal plane plantarflexion from TA	
Type 3 (Sangeorzan)	Body 3A: coronal 3B: dorsolateral—>plantarmedial (major medial frag) 3C comminution (major lateral frag)	3B: adduction 3C: abduction	
Type 4	Stress fracture	running	• occurs usually at plantar-central avascular region • **acute injury** (low sclerosis on CT): percutaneous • **chronic injury** (high sclerosis on CT): graft

DX:
- **XR:** multiple views due to possible obliquity of fracture
- **MRI, bone scan, CT:** for stress fracture
- test PTT muscle strength

TX: NWB!!!! in cast

Calcaneal fracture, calcaneus fracture

MC of all tarsal bone fractures!

Challenges:
- complex articular anatomy

134

- subcutaneous lateral wall
- limited areas of dense bone, (except thalamic portion under posterior facet, sustentaculum tali, and apex of the angle of Gissane (lateral aspect of sinus tarsi)
- sharply sloping medial wall with its closed associated soft tissue structures

ET: fall from height with axial load, forcing foot into varus position

CP:
- Mondor's sign-plantar ecchymosis
- Back pain (20%), between T12 and L2 (L1 most common)
  - Rule out peroneal subluxation!!!
- Compartment syndrome (15% due to excessive bleeding from calcaneus)
  - Hoffa's sign-less taut Achilles tendon
  - Lateral wall blowout-when posterior facet driven down body of calcaneus

DX:
- urinalysis to r/o urinary trauma
- XR, CT

CT: coronal view, gold standard for surgical planning

XR:
- foot, LUMBAR + PELVIC XR
- Broden's view-to view POSTERIOR facet
  - knee flexed, foot internally rotated 45 degrees, 10, 20, 30, 40 cephalic tilt to view anterior—>posterior portions of posterior facet
- Isherwood view-3 oblique views to view ALL facets
- Calcaneal Axial view-lateral widening and varus orientation

Calcaneal radiographic angles

	Normal	Calcaneal fx	Formed by
Bohler's angle	20-40	DECREASED	Calcaneal tuberosity, posterior facet, anterior beak
Gissane's angle or critical/crucial angle	120-145	INCREASED	Posterior facet, anterior shelf

	Rowe	Articular	Freq	Other	Sanders
1A	Medial tuberosity	extra-articular	20%		NON-DISPLACED (lateral)
1B	Sustentaculum tali	extra-articular	20%	pain with hallux ROM	NON-DISPLACED (middle)
1C	Anterior process	extra-articular	20%	PF inversion injury with bifurcate ligament avulsion	NON-DISPLACED (medial)
2A	Posterior process	extra-articular	20%		DISPLACED (lateral)
2B	Posterior @ Achilles insertion (Beak fracture)	extra-articular	20%		DISPLACED (middle)
2C					DISPLACED (medial)
3	Oblique body	extra-articular	20%		

					3 fragments
3AB, 3AC, 3BC					
4	Oblique body	intra-articular	60%	Surgery	Comminuted with 4+ fragments
5	Comminuted/jt depression	intra-articular	60%	Surgery	

Rowe Classification, Sanders Classification
Essex Lopresti Classification
- Extra articular-25%
-
    Intra-articular-75%, A and B type
    o <u>Primary fracture line:</u> vertical fracture line due to talus eversion, driving lateral process into Gissane's angle, through neutral triangle

	Type	Secondary fracture line	MOA
A	Tongue type	Extending posteriorly proximal to Achilles insertion	force directed **inferior** to posterior facet
B	Joint depression	Driven down cancellous bone of body of calcaneus	force directed **through** posterior facet

Fragments

Fragment	Description
Superomedial	constant fragment, under sustentaculum tali to which all others are fixed
Anterolateral	
Lateral	Essex lopresti A-"thalamic" or "comet fragment", under posterior facet Essex lopresti B-"semilunar fragment"
Tuberosity	displaced varus and laterally

TX:
Conservative: Air cast, CAM boot
- Poor outcome when having to convert to triple arthrodesis, compared to initial ORIF
- **For displaced intra-articular fractures, NO DIFFERENCE compared to surgery at 3 year follow up (Sutherland, Cochrane 2013[125])**

Surgical (ORIF):
- Within 12 hours before acute swelling begins
    o After swelling resides (7-10 days s/p injury), within 2 weeks before hematoma organization
    o Lateral extensile approach
        o Caution lateral calcaneal branch of peroneal artery (LCBP)
        o subcutaneous nature of lateral calcaneal wall increases risk for wound dehiscence
        o Donati Allgower stitch
    o 1) Tuberosity fragment 2) restore posterior facet height 3) reduce lateral wall blow-out
    o **Shantz pin:** 1) bring tuberosity out to length by applying traction force 2) values position 3) translate medially
        o keep NWB x 8 wks

Goals:

---

[125] Bruce J, Sutherland A. Cochrane Database Syst Rev. 2013 Jan 31;1:CD008628.

- Restore height/length
- Prevent varus/valgus tilt
- Prevent posterior facet step-off

Procedure	Indications	Complications
ORIF	severe sander's (comminuted) fracture, Bohler angle <0, worker's comp, heavy laborers (Buckley JBJS 2002[126])	can —> STJ arthritis requiring STJ fusion
STJ fusion	severely comminuted displaced intra-calcaneal fracture Bohler angle <0	

Complications: wound healing, ankle impingement, nonunion

Podiatric surgical emergency:
- Gas gangrene
- Open fracture/dislocation
- Compartment syndrome
  - Necrotizing fasciitis

Shock
Hypovolemic,
Cardiogenic-inability for heart to pump
Septic
Anaphylactic-excess release of histamine which causes widespread vasodilation
Neurogenic-damage to spinal cord results in loss of autonomic/motor reflexes
Obstructive-obstruction of circulation

Gustillo Anderson Classification for Open fracture

Stage	Description	How to close wound	Infxn rate	ABx*
1	Wound < 1 cm	primary closure	0-2%	1st gen cephalosporin (Ancef)
2	Wound 1-5cm, no XS soft tissue damage	primary closure	2-7%	Ancef, clindamycin
3	Wound >5cm + soft tissue damage (mm, skin, neurovascular structures)	delayed primary closure (DPC)	10-25%	Ancef, clindamycin, aminoglycoside (gram -)
3A	Soft tissue covering adequate		7%	
3B	Excess soft tissue loss		10-50%	
3C	Arterial injury (call vascular surgeon!)		25-50%	

*add millions of units of PCN for anaerobic (farm) injuries
    - Risk for compartment syndrome
    - INFECTED when untreated for 6-8 hours
TX:
- tetanus and NV status

[126] Buckley, Richard, et al. "Operative compared with nonoperative treatment of displaced intra-articular calcaneal fractures." *The Journal of Bone & Joint Surgery* 84.10 (2002): 1733-1744.

- Culture and sensitivity
- Incision and drainage

Goals:
- Prevent infection
- Blood flow within 6 hours
- Start ABx immediately
- Debride using I&D, repeat @ 24, 72 hours

Fracture blisters

ET:
- Due to high energy trauma mechanical shear force: calcaneal, ankle, Lisfranc fracture
  - Edema 2/2 interstitial pressure
- Typically 24-48 hours post injury
- Early operation prevents formation of blisters

CP:
> Sub-epidermal
>   - Fluid filled-more common (75%)
>   - Blood filled-more severe

TX:
  - Risk infection, vascular compromise, skin healing issue
- Best to wait for blister to resolve rather than cutting through it

Compartment Syndrome
Bleeding/edema in a closed nonelastic muscle compartment surrounded by fascia or bone, closing off blood supply

ET:
  - Crush injury (calcaneus), high-energy deceleration trauma—> increased compartment pressure —> venous HTN to prevent vascular collapse—>microcirculation shuts down
  - muscle necrosis @ 3 hours

DX:
  - Stryker (Wick's), slit catheter
- Positive test:
- Intracompartmental pressure > 30 mmHg (normal 0-5mmHg)
- Compartment pressure within 10-30mmHg of diastolic BP

CP: 6P's: pain out of proportion (most sensitive), parasthesia, pallor, pulselessness (least sensitive), paresis, paralysis, pressure.
- more common in leg than foot
Volkman's contracture-ischemic necrosis causes muscle contracture
- 9 compartments: superficial and deep central, medial, 4 interosseeus, lateral plantar, deep interosseus

Compartment	Contents
Medial	abductor hallucis, FHB
Central	FDB, lumbricals, QP, adductor hallucis, FDL, PTT, PL
Lateral	Abductor digiti minimi, flexor digiti minimi
Interosseus	

TX: Fasciotomy
- within 8-12 hrs of injury before irreversible nerve/muscle damage
- incision over 2nd, 4th MT

Chronic exertional compartment syndrome
Overuse condition in young athletes causing exercise-related pain
- Mostly anterior compartment of leg

Tetanus

ET: open wound >6 hrs,
CP: triad: trismus (lockjaw), risus sardonicus (spastic facial muscle), aphagia
TX:
Known booster: 0.5cc of toxoid IM within last 5 years
Unknown booster: toxoid + 250mg immuglobulin IM

Puncture wound

Origin	Organism
most common OM, or through shoe	pseudomonas
soil	clostridia
dog bite	pasturella multocida, capnocytophaga canimorsus, strep viridans
cat bite	pasturella multocida
cat scratch	bartonella henslae (cat scratch fever)
human bite	eikenella, strep viridans

Digital Fractures, bedpost fracture
CP: hallux MC fracture, more specifically proximal phalanx
Rosenthal Classification

Zone	Description	Treatment
Zone 1	Distal to distal aspect of distal phalanx	
Zone 2	Distal to lunula	**Atasoy flap**-plantar V-Y **Kutler flap**-biaxial V-Y
Zone 3	Distal to most distal joint	distal Symes

Pediatric Pathology

Clubfoot, congenital talipes equinovarus (CTEV), talipes equinovarus (TEV)
"Talipes" = adduction of TALUS 80-90 degrees (normal 15-20)
ET/RF:
  1) **Idiopathic**, one of the most common MSK birth defects
     a. malposition of talar head and neck
     b. Myelomeningiocele, oligohydramnios
  2) **Acquired**-NM disorder, arthrogryphosis, spina bifida
CP:
  • **AVE: forefoot ADDUCTION + hindfoot VARUS + EQUINUS**
  • 0 degree talocalcaneal angle
  • **Empty heel sign**-unable to palpate calcaneus posteriorly
  • Cavus: walking on side/top of feet, callus formation
DX:
- CC angle
- Kite's angle <15 (normal 18, 20-40), more superimposed
- CIA
- **Horizontal breech**-bimalleolar axis <75 (angle between AP bisection of hindfoot and malleolar plane) is indicative of clubfoot
- **Beatson and pearson**-AP talocalc + lateral talocalc <40 is indicative of clubfoot

- **Simon's rule of 15**-AP talo-1st MT angle >15 is indicative of clubfoot

TX:

Gold standard: Ponseti manipulation and casting + Achilles tenotomy
- o   Start within first few weeks of life
- o   5-7 serial casts
- o   Foot abduction bracing up to 4 y.o.
- o   monitor CC angle
- o   **Casting risks**: AVN of talar head, dorsal subluxation of navicular on talar head
- •   French/functional method
- •   Surgery has poor results in adulthood
- •   **Surgical indication**: rigid deformity, NM etiology,

Pediatric fracture

Salter-Harris classification

	Description
1	through growth plate
2 *	above, MOST COMMON: Thurston Holland sign "Flag sign", fragment extending from growth plate
3 *	below
4	Through AKA **triplane fracture**
5	crush
6	Physis injury, bony bridge, angular deformity
7	epiphyseal plate
8	metaphyseal injury with endochondral ossification
9	periosteum injury

**Salter 2&3 are "triplanar fx"

TX:

Fixation for physeal fracture: K wire

Talipes calcaneovalgus (TCV) aka flexible pes planovalgus

CP: XS calcaneal DF-dorsum of foot touches anterior shin, valgus, flexible flatfoot

MOST INFANTS ARE FLATFOOTED AND DEVELOP ARCH DURING 1ST DECADE OF LIFE

TX: stretch posterior compartment, casting, spontaneous resolution

Developmental dislocation (dysplasia) of hip (DDH)

CP:

Anchor's sign-asymmetry of thigh and and gluteal folds (more folds on dislocated side)

Galeazzi's sign-with knee bent, lower knee position

Trendelenburg-standing on affected side causes normal side of hip to drop

DX:

Barlow's test-dislocates unstable hip

Ortolani test-relocation of a dislocated hip. Abduct hip —> click—> + post dislocation of hip. Tests for dislocatable hip

TX: Pavlik harness-for newborns

Congenital vertical talus (CVT), convex pes planovalgus, Persian slipper foot

Dorsal dislocation of navicular on talar neck with talus in vertical position.

ET: bone, tendon, capsule, soft tissue abnormality.

CP:
- congenital rocker bottom
- RIGIDITY: lack of motion at STJ/ankle joint
- ABducted foot, DF at MTJ with dislocated TN joint
- Heel valgus, equinus
- majority b/l
- **Peg leg gait**, limited FF push off
- Contraction of TA, EHL, EDL, peroneal tendons
    - Negative calcaneal inclination angle
    - **Arthrogryphosis** (multiple joint contractures)
    o Delayed walking, plantar callus 2/2 talar head

DX: XR: lateral view-***hourglass*** talar neck

TX:

Conservative: CANNOT cast due to rigid deformity

Surgical:
- ORIF TNJ with k-wire (1-4 yo)
- **Green Grice procedure**-extra articular arthrodesis of STJ (4-6 yo)
- Triple arthrodesis (>12 yo)
- Arthroeresis, talectomy, removal of navicular

Muscular dystrophies

	Duchenne	Beckers	Fascio-scapulohumeral
Genetic etiology	Absent dystrophin, sex-linked recessive	Altered dystrophin	
Clinical presentation	Pseudohypertrophy-apparent hypertrophy of muscle, not fat Equinus, toe walking with IQ drop, Gower's sign, waddling gait. Die at age 20	Similar to Duchenne with no IQ drop, Cavovarus foot	Popeye arms
Age	5	40	
Diagnosis	Muscle biopsy and muscle strength evaluation	Same as duchenne	

Metatarsus adductus, met adductus, MT adductus

ET:
- intrauterine position
- tight abductor hallucis
- most likely 2/2 to tibial torsion or femoral anteversion (externally rotated hips)

EP: 1 in 1000 live births

CP:
- Flexible, rigid, or dynamic-congenitally normal foot becomes C-shaped due to contracture of abductor hallucis
- "C-shaped foot"
- Intoeing, shoe not fitting, tripping, 5th MT styloid process pain, compensatory overpronation
- **Positive V-finger test**: lateral border curves away from middle finger starting at 5th MT styloid process
- Compensation: pronation at STJ

Bleck	Bisection of heel
Normal	between 2nd/3rd
Mild	thru 3rd
Moderate	between 3rd/4th
Severe	between 4th/5th

Bleck Classification: Radiograph:
- Engel's angle (2nd MT and intermediate cuneiform)
    - Simon's angle: bisection of talar neck and 1st MT

NH:
- 90% correct by 3 months
- 4% remain by 16 y.o.

TX:

Conservative (<3 y.o.)	Soft tissue procedure (3-8 y.o.)	Osseus procedure (>8 y.o.)
-**Gold std: Manipulation + serial casting** -Ganley splint- triplanar correction -Unibar -Dennis Brown Bar	-Abductor hallucis release -**Heyman, Herndon, Strong (HHS procedure)**- capsulotomy of TMT and intercuneiform ligaments EXCEPT lateral and plantar lateral ligaments -**Thompson**-abductor hallucis resection -TATT -Medial midfoot capsulotomy -Thompson-resect abductor hallucis, medial head FHB if necessary	-**Berman and Gartland:** lateral crescentic osteotomies of MT base 1-5 -OBWO of medial cuneiform + CBWO of cuboid -Johnson osteochondrotomy-closing ABductory wedge -**Lepird:** oblique rotational osteotomies of MT 2-5, CBWO of MT 1 & 5

Skewfoot, skewfoot deformity (SFD), complex metatarsus adductus, compensated metatarsus adductus, metatarsus associated flatfoot, congenital metatarsus varus, serpentine foot, Z foot, complex skewfoot
CP:
MT adductus + rearfoot valgus
- Adducted FF, normal midfoot, valgus RF
    - HPK over PF'd talus
- congenital rocker bottom

DX:
- LATERAL displacement of navicular on talar head
- **Complex MT adductus**: MT add, midfoot medial translation
- **Simple skewfoot**: MT add, normal midfoot, RF valgus
- **Complex skewfoot**: MT add, lateral midfoot, RF valgus

TX:
- wait until early childhood
- soft tissue and osseous procedures

Generalized joint hypermobility (GJH), joint hypermobility syndrome (JHS)
- Beighton score is a useful instrument to evaluate school aged children 6-12 years old

Brachymetatarsia
RF: Down syndrome, Turner's, hyperPTH, polio
CP:
- >5mm short
- 4th MT most common, then 1st MT

TX:
- One step lengthening when target length <1.5cm
Gradual lengthening when target length >1.5cm
Corticotomy (leave only medullary vv) and callus distraction
- Max is 1.5cm due to neuromuscular stretching!!!
- Adjunct V-Y skin plasty or Z-plasty for EDL tendon
Calculate callus distraction time: compress x 7 days, distract 1mm per day MAX, then wait 2x amount of distraction time. i.e. to lengthen 5mm: 7 + 5 + 10 = 22

Syndactyly
CP: MC congenital deformity

Radiology

Angle of gait:
>   Amount foot deviates from line of progression
>   7-10 degrees

Base of gait:
>   Distance between medial malleoli
>   ~1 inch

AP radiograph:
- Beam 15 degrees from perpendicular, in cephalad direction
- Aim for MTJ (base of 3rd MT)
- Patient facing direction of progression

Lateral radiograph:
- Foot parallel to film
- Contralateral foot in angle and base of gait

Oblique:
1) tube at 35 degrees
2) Medial oblique (foot planted on medial surface)
    a. view the cuboid, navicular, lateral foot
3) Lateral oblique

Hindfoot Alignment view
- Beam at 10 degrees, film at 10 degrees
- Measure distance between line perpendicular to bisection of tibia and lowest point of calcaneus
>   To measure RF coronal plane axis

Calcaneal axial view
>   posterior calcaneus, to visualize calcaneal trauma

Dorsoplantar: tube 25 degrees from vertical, patient in ski jump position

Plantodorsal: tube at 40-45 degrees from vertical. Patient in supine position. Heel placed against cassette, and toes point upward. The patient forcibly dorsiflexes the forefoot.

Harris Beath aka Coalition view
>   Views medal and posterior STJ facets (useful for talocalcaneal coalition)
>   same as DP calcaneal axial except tube 35-45 degrees

Broden view
>   Ankle DF'ed, leg internally rotated 30 degrees
>   XR beam with cephalic tilt 10-40 degrees

Ankle mortise view
>   AP view with 15 deg internal rotation
>   parallel lines <4mm

Cyma line
>   Anterior break (pronated) —TN joint over CC
>   Posterior break (supinated) –TN joint posterior to CC

longitudinal bisection of	region of foot	measurement
tarsus	rearfoot	Line parallel to the lateral border of calcaneus, anterior superior medial calcaneus on AP view
lesser tarsus	midfoot	Line used in MAA

---

[127] Radiology and Biomechanical Foot Types, Donald R. Green, Podiatry Institute Update, 1998

longitudinal bisection of	region of foot	measurement
2nd MT	forefoot	bisect 2nd MT

Forefoot adductus angle
> Angle formed by forefoot and rearfoot (2nd MT to RF angle)
> Normally slightly less than MAA
>> low FFA and high MAA indicates pronated foot

Lesser tarsus abductus angle AKA lesser tarsus angle
> Angle formed by rearfoot and midfoot
> Positional angle

Metatarsus adductus angle (MAA)
> Angle formed by forefoot and midfoot
> MOST IMPORTANT ANGLE TO DETERMINE TRANSVERSE PLANE FOOT STRUCTURE (adducted vs rectus foot)

Lesser tarsus abductus angle
> Angle formed by midfoot and rearfoot

Cuboid abduction angle
> Lateral border of cuboid with rearfoot angle

Tibial sesamoid position
> 1-7
> Position 4 is centered over bisection of 1st MT

Tibial sesamoid 2nd MT distance (TSMD)
> Angle formed by line perpendicular to tibial sesamoid and line down 2nd MT

1st MT calcaneus angle
> relationship of compensated position of 1st MT to foot
>> can mask high IMA or high MAA
> estimation of transverse deviation of 1st MT from the rear foot
> takes into account structural MAA and forefoot adductus angle

Calcaneal inclination angle (CIA)
> Proximal plantar surface to anterior-inferior CC joint compared to WB surface
> NOT altered by pronation/supination

Kirby's sign
> Posterior facet of talus abuts calcaneal floor and occludes sinus tarsi
> Sign of maximum pronation
> Opposite of bullet hole sinus tarsi

Talo-1st MT angle (Meary's angle)
> Positive-DF of first ray on TN segment
>> Unstable 1st MT
> Negative-PF of first raty on TN segment
>> Stability of 1st ray on FF

Seiberg index
> Used to dx MPE
> Relationship of sagittal plane of 1st MT to 2nd MT
> DISTAL — PROXIMAL:

Positive = MPE
Negative = no MPE
[Distance from dorsum of 2nd MT neck to 1st MT neck] — [Distance from dorsum of 2nd MT shaft to 1st MT shaft 1.5cm from articular base]

Angles

Angle	Pes planus	Pes cavus	Normal, positional vs structural
Kite's (AP talocalcaneal) (long. bisection of calc + bisect of talar head and neck)	30-50 (inc) RF VALGUS	<15 (dec)	18 (20-40)
Cuboid abduction angle aka calcaneocuboid angle	>5 (inc)	<0 (dec)	0-5
Lateral talocalcaneal (CIA + TDA)	Increased	Decreased	45
Calcaneal inclination (CIA) / Calcaneal pitch	10-18 mod <10 severe	30-40 mod >40 severe	18-30 Avg: 24.5 (structural)
Talar declination angle (TDA)	Increased	Decreased	21
Meary's (lateral talo-1st MT)	Positive **(NC fault)** (hypermobile 1st ray)	Negative (stable 1st ray)	0
1st MT declination angle	DECREASED	INCREASED	19-25 combined
Seiberg index (distal - proximal)	Increased (positive, MPE)	Decreased (PF 1st ray)	combined
Hibb's (calcaneo-1st MT)		<150	>150
Cyma line	Anterior break	Posterior break	positional
Talar head covering aka talonavicular congruity	<3/4	>3/4	>3/4
Lesser tarsus abductus angle aka **lesser tarsus angle** (midfoot to rearfoot)	Increase	Decrease	Positional
Forefoot adductus angle (2nd MT to rearfoot)	DECREASED	INCREASED	0-10 positional
1st MT calcaneal angle (estimates 1st MT deviation from RF)	DECREASED	INCREASED	combined

Sinus tarsi	Kirby's sign	Bullet hole	
Superimposition of MT	Increased	Decreased	
TN/NC fault	Yes		
DF talus	Yes		
Navicular height	Decrease	Increase	
5th MT declincation	Increased	Decreased	combined
Angle of Gissane (crucial angle)- anterior process to sulcus to posterior facet			120-140
Bohler's angle-posterior facet to calcaneal tuberosity			25-40
Fowler Philip Angle			<75

Bunion angles	Structural vs positional	Normal	Abnormal
HAA angle o increases with hypermobile 1st ray	combined	15-16	Mild: 15-20 Moderate: 20-40 Severe: >40
HIA angle		<10	>10
PASA (1st MT articular surface vs shaft)	adaptation of cartilaginous surface of 1st MT head	7.5 (similar to HAA)	>8
DASA (prox phalanx articular surface vs shaft)	lateral deviation of shaft of proximal phalanx	7.5 (not a good measurement)	>8
Met adductus angle (MAA)	structural	10-20, 15	
Engel's angle (bisection of 2nd MT and intermed cuneiform) *Quick estimation for MAA*	structural	<18	
Simon's angle (assess met adductus) (talar neck and 1st MT)		<20	>20
Intermetatarsal angle (IMA) aka metatarsus primus adducts (increases with hypermobile 1st ray)	structural	<8	Mild 8-12 Moderate: 12-15 Severe: >15
True IMA: IMA + (MAA – 15)	structural	8-10 measure only when MAA > 15	

146

	combined	1-3	>3 (4 is @ bisection of 1st MT)
Tibial sesamoid position (TSP)			
Fallat and Buckholz angle (4th MT and medial cortex)		<7 (2.64)	8.05
5th MT IMA		<7 (6.47)	8.71
Lateral deviation angle (LDA) aka lateral bowing angle (5th MT head & medial cortex)		3	>8
MT protrusion distance		+/- 2mm	

Ankle Radiographs

	Ligament	Positive test
Anterior drawer test	ATFL	Displacement of 1 cm or >3mm than other side
Valgus talar tilt test	Deltoid	>10 degrees +/- 6-8 deg
Varus talar tilt test	CFL/ATFL	>10 degrees
Laxity with PF/inversion	ATFL	
Laxity with DF/inversion	CFL	
Mortise radiograph/Medial clear space	Deltoid	>4mm
Tibia fibula clear space	Syndesmosis	>6mm
External rotation stress view	Deltoid	>5mm
Talocrural angle		8-15, +/- 2-5 deg of other side

How to read XR
- **Overall Overview**
  o labeled (name, age), marker R/L
  o Exposure
  o Views
  o WB/NWB
  o Quality
- **Soft tissue**
  o density, foreign body, calcifications, contour, gas/emphysema, defects, tumors/mass, artifacts
- **Bone**
  o cortex integrity, thickness of cortex, density, periosteal reaction, erosions, bone tumor/masses, fractures, subchondral sclerosis, physeal plates, morphology, quantity
- **Joints**
  o subchondral sclerosis, width, congruency, position, loose bodies/joint mice, coalition, orientation
- **Biomechanical (WB ONLY)**
  o joint deformities, angles

Soft tissue: soft tissue density/contour, gas, vascular calcification, foreign body, break in cortices
Cavus/Planus:
  1. (everything decreases in cavus, everything increases in planus EXCEPT talar head covering, 1st MT declination, 1st MT calc, navicular height)

Lateral: CIA, lateral talocalcaneal angle (dec/inc), talar declination (dec/inc), Meary's (dec/inc), Kirby's sign, Cyma line, superimposition of MT (dec/inc), 1st MT declination (INC/DEC)
AP: MAA, Kite's (dec/inc), cuboid abduction (dec/inc), talar head covering (INC/DEC)

HAV:
AP: MAA, Kite's, FFAA, talar uncovering, cuboid abduction, IMA moderately elevated, HAA moderately elevated, TSP, PASA/DASA mildly elevated, HIA within normal limits, 1st MT protrusion

Flatfoot
Lateral: CIA decreased, (lateral talocalaneal angle increased), talar declination angle increased, 1st MT declination angle DECREASED, Meary's angle increased, Kirby's sign present, anterior break in cyma line, increased superimposition of metatarsals, elevated 1st Metatarsal due to positive Seiberg index

Biomechanics

Biomechanics[128]
- Motion can occurs in a plane <u>perpendicular</u> to the joint axis
- Motion DOES NOT occur in an axis that it is <u>parallel</u> to (can be two planes)
- <u>Translational equilibrium</u>: ground reactive forces (GRF) are equal and opposite to the loading force (forces involved in the ankle joint)
- <u>Rotational equilibrium</u>: seesaw analogy (a dorsiflexed forefoot vs tension at the Achilles tendon)
- GRF through forefoot combined with tensile strength at Achilles means compression force at ankle joint at least 3x body weight[129]

Biomechanical exam
- Prone position:
  - draw line to bisect calcaneus using two thumbs
  - determine amount of inversion/eversion relative to achilles
  - have patient DF to determine equinus
  - determine FF to RF relationship when putting foot in STJ neutral
- Standing:
  - re-draw bisection of calcaneus as the skin might have moved with weight bearing
  - have patient invert and evert from standing position to determine if they are in a maximally pronated/supinated position

Standing exam
- Eyes, head, neck face position
- Shoulder/UE symmetry
- Spine linearity
- Hip symmetry
- Knee alignment
- Tibia alignment
- Midfoot position: RCSP/NCSP
- Forefoot position: RCSP/NCSP
- Base of gait
- Digital position/windlass mechanism

Gait evaluation
- Eyes, face, head, neck, shoulder symmetry
- Arm swing
- Spine linearity

[128] Seibel, Michael O. Foot Function: A programmed text. Williams & Wilkins, 1988
[129] Stauffer, Richard N., Edward YS Chao, and Robert C. Brewster. "Force and motion analysis of the normal, diseased, and prosthetic ankle joint." Clinical orthopaedics and related research 127 (1977): 189-196.

- Hip alignment, symmetry
- Knee
- Tibia
- Rearfoot
- Midfoot
- Forefoot
- Line of progression
- Angle and base of gait
- Overall type of gait

Gait cycle
- 1 cycle: heel strike of one foot —> heel strike of same foot

STANCE (HEEL STRIKE —> FF LOADING —> HEEL LIFT —> TOE OFF) —> SWING

STANCE 60% (heel strike —> toe off)

	Start/end	Actions	Ratio
1. Contact	Heel strike to forefoot loading	STJ **pronation** *"mobile adaptor", "loose bag of bones", "unlocked", shock absorption*	30%
2. Midstance*	Forefoot loading to toe off	STJ **supination** *"rigid lever", "MTJ locked", "close-packed position", maximum efficiency*	40%
3. Propulsion	Toe off to heel strike	STJ **supination** (foot is *rigid lever*), maximum efficiency gliding of 1st MT head over sesamoid apparatus Abnormal pronation would cause *hypermobility*	30%

In relation to other foot:
- Contact: **Heel strike** of same foot to toe off of opposite foot
- Midstance: Toe off of opposite foot to **heel lift** of same foot
- Propulsion: **Heel lift** of same foot to **toe off** of same foot

SWING 40% (toe off —> heel strike)

	Motion	Function
First half	OKC pronation	helps foot clear ground
Second half	OKC supination	stabilizes foot to prepare for heel strike

*Peroneus longus
- Retrograde resupination when tendon fires:
    - plantarflexes/everts 1st ray,
    - stabilizes medial column,
    - locks the MTJ
    - works in tandem with plantar fascia
- opposes medial deviation of 1st MT
- fires during midstance —> propulsion phase of gait
    - increased activity in flat-footed individuals
    - prepares for windlass mechanism to take effect
- Rectus foot (navicular superior to cuboid):

149

- o good function, holds 1st ray rigid
- Pronated foot (navicular inferior to cuboid)
  - o poor function, P. longus now parallel to ground —> increased 1st ray hypermobility

Open vs closed kinetic chain (OKC vs CKC) of STJ motion
STJ pronation:
1. abduction, eversion, and DF of the calcaneus (and foot) on the talus (and leg) OR
   - *Calcaneus: eversion, abduction, DF*
2. adduction, inversion, and PF of the talus (and leg) on the calcaneus (and foot)
   - *Talus: inversion, adduction, PF*

OKC: movement around a joint that is NWB-calcaneus moves around talus, which acts as extension of leg
CKC: Both calcaneus and talus move

	OKC Pronation	OKC Supination	CKC Pronation	CKC Supination
calcaneus	eversion	inversion	eversion	inversion
talus (transverse plane)	abduction	adduction	adduction	abduction
talus (saggittal plane)	DF	PF	PF	DF
tibia (follows talus)			internal rotation	external rotation

Direction STJ moves towards	Increased deformity in what plane?
more vertical position	transverse plane
more transverse position	frontal plane
more parallel to frontal plane	saggital plane

Subtalar joint (STJ):
- Most movement in FRONTAL plane
- Motion in <u>sagittal</u> and <u>transverse</u> plane
  - o 16 degrees from sagittal (Sixteen = Sagittal)
  - o 42 degrees from transverse (forty Two = Transverse)
- Direction: proximal lateral plantar (PLP)—>distal medial dorsal (DMD)
  - o Posterior calcaneus —> anterior talar neck
- STJ ROM: 30° total
  - o 2/3 supination (INV) 20°
  - o 1/3 pronation (EV) 10°

STJ neutral position
- The point where bisection of posterior calcaneus is parallel to bisection distal 1/3 of leg
- The position in which STJ neither pronated/supinated
- The point where inversion and eversion of calcaneus will purely be in the frontal plane, free of transverse/sagittal plane motion
- Neutral: the position of a joint in which maximal ROM can occur in either direction

Calculating STJ neutral:
- STJ neutral = [(INV + EV) / 3] – EV
- (add any tibial varum/valgum)*
- Calculate total STJ ROM, calculate normal expected INV/EV, and compare with actual values

- ○ Negative = EVERTED, STJ valgus
- ○ Positive = INVERTED, STJ varus

*The amount of compensation requires adding the tibial component (7 deg eversion, 2 deg tibial varum = 9 deg pronatory compensation)

Causes of STJ pronation

RF varus	additional pronation required during compensation, cannot catch up during resupination. Foot remains supinated —> loose bag of bones —> hyper mobility
equinus	foot pronates to compensate for PF'ed foot
RF valgus	compensation results in more pronation. Foot remains pronated through entire gait cycle
tarsal coalition	results in RF valgus

MTJ:
- • 2 axes:
- • Longitudinal and oblique axis
- • Oblique
  - ○ **Sagittal/transverse** plane motion
  - ○ PF = adduction, DF = abduction ("PAD DAB")
- • Longitudinal
  - ○ **Frontal** plane motion

MTJ affected by STJ.
1. *"STJ is the key, MTJ is the lock: STJ in neutral, with MTJ maximally pronated, locked position"*

STJ position	MTJ position	result at MTJ	result at medial column
supinated	oblique to each other (pronated)*	locked MTJ, ROM restricted	stable medial column
pronated	parallel to each other (supinated)	unlocked MTJ, increased ROM	hypermobile first ray

*MTJ maximally pronated, locked position: plantar plates of FF and RF are parallel with each other
1. THIS IS THE BASIS OF ASSESSING THE FOREFOOT TO REARFOOT RELATIONSHIP

	full compensation	partial compensation
forefoot varus*	</= 2 degrees, STJ pronates —> RECTUS	>/= 3 degrees, STJ **pronates to end ROM****
forefoot valgus	LA SOS Longitudinal Axis of MTJ inverts STJ supinates Oblique axis of MTJ pronates STJ supinates	

	full compensation	partial compensation
forefoot supinatus	fixed inverted forefoot position due to soft tissue adaptation 2/2 to flatfoot with RF valgus	

*Because FF varus always compensates by pronation, will need a RF VARUS post in orthotic
** Maximally pronated STJ "to end range of motion": lateral facet of talus hits the floor of the sinus tarsi. Interosseus compression of sinus tarsi can increase as the foot continues to pronate. This can lead to sinus tarsi syndrome

First ray axis:

OPPOSITE OF STJ!!!

    Motion: 45 degrees from <u>frontal</u> and <u>sagittal</u> plane
        5mm Dorsiflexion, Inversion (Siebel)
        5mm Plantarflexion, Eversion (Siebel)
    Axis: <u>transverse</u> plane
    Metatarsus primus elevatus:
            DF > PF
            leads to hyper mobility of medial column
            hallux rigidus
    Plantarflexed first ray
            PF > DF
    Hypermobility/1st ray insufficiency:
            1st ray insufficiency is the symptom of a hypermobile first ray.
            Results in shearing forces, joint subluxation, fatigue, hyperkeratotic callus
            Hypermobile means 1st ray is moving when it should be stable
            <u>Windlass mechanism</u>-DF hallux increases arch of foot
            <u>Reverse windlass mechanism</u>-a lowered arch results in a PF hallux. Windlass unable to overcome ground reactive
                force on first ray. Foot is unable to resupinate.
            Greater space/diastasis @ Lisfranc's joint may indicate hypermobility
            Medial deviation of STJ prevents the windlass mechanism from engaging
            Greater DF of 1st ray results in less 1st MTPJ DF (Roukis)
            Equinus
                overload of forefoot
                instability of peroneus longus
                foot pronates to allow for greater dorsiflexion in mid foot
                heel plantigrade

5th ray axis:
    Same as STJ

Central 3 rays, IPJ, MPJ axis:
    Motion in <u>sagittal</u> plane

Normal foot:
    Distal 1/3 leg vertical
    Knee, ankle, STJ parallel to transverse plane of ground
    Vertical bisection of calcaneus
    MTJ maximally pronated

Hip:
    Normal ROM is 45 degrees internal/external rotation
Femoral version
    Bisection of femoral head & neck
        Birth: 30-35
        Adult: 10-12

	Anteversion	Retroversion
Femur position	Posterior to frontal plane of body	Anterior to frontal plane of body
Hip position	EXTERNALLY rotated	INTERNALLY rotated

Femoral inclination

	Coxa Vara	Coxa Valga
Angle of femoral inclination	< 128 degrees	>128 degrees
Etiology	femoral head dysplasia	slipped capital femoral epiphysis, trauma
Concurrent knee	genu valgum (knock knee)	genu varum (bow legged)

Ontogeny

	At birth	At maturity (4-6 y.o.)	Rotation
Femoral torsion (twist)	30 degrees internally rotated	10 degrees internally rotated	External rotation of distal femur
Femoral version (rotate)	60 degrees anteversion (externally rotated)	10 degrees anteversion	Internal rotation of proximal femur

Ankle joint axis
- Mostly sagittal plane
  - **83 degrees from coronal plane**
  - **23 degrees from transverse plane**
  - (or: 8 degrees from transverse, 16 degrees from frontal, 82 degrees from sagittal)

CKC

Angle of gait: angle of feet relative to body's line of progression during gait
Base of gait: closest width between malleoli during midstance
NCSP aka rearfoot varus/valgus:
  WB exam
  STJ neutral + tibial varum/valgum.
  Determines rearfoot varus/valgus

	Etiology	Full compensation	Partial compensation

	Etiology	Full compensation	Partial compensation
RF varus *calculate total amount of eversion by adding eversion and STJ neutral value*	rickets (vitamin D deficiency), Blounts disease (medial metaphyseal lesion), femoral/knee/tibial abnormalities	STJ pronation until deformity returns perpendicular to ground	calcaneus still in inverted position
RF valgus	tarsal coalition (peroneal spastic flatfoot)	If NCSP greater than/equal 3 deg, will drive to end ROM: RCSP: total eversion – amount of tibial varum	If NCSP less than/equal 2 deg, no compensation, RCSP = NCSP

RCSP (compensated rearfoot varus/valgus):
    NCSP plus amount of compensation.
Fully compensated : RCSP perpendicular to ground with NCSP in varus/valgus

Subtalar varus/valgus: in STJ neutral, calcaneus inversion/eversion **relative to distal 1/3 of leg**
Rearfoot varus/valgus: in STJ neutral, calcaneus inversion/eversion **relative to ground**

	Tibial bowing	Effect on calcaneus
Tibial varum/genu varum	Inward	Inversion
Tibial valgum/genu valgum	Outward	Eversion

Rearfoot pathology
STJ pronation during propulsion: equinus and rearfoot varus

Orthotics
    Although under the STJ, redirects the ground reactive forces acting on the plantar foot in a medial direction to cause foot to supinate
    Works just like the T-strap brace which produces a medial directing force AT the STJ

	Contributions	Definition of Pathology
Root theory (1958)	-"Father of podiatric biomechanics" -Modern thermoplastic foot orthoses -8 biophysical criteria for normalcy -STJ neutral position to lock MTJ, prevent compensation -STJ neutral suspension casting -does not apply mechanical and WB behavior of foot	-Deviation in STJ causes pronation and supination due to ground reactive forces. -Orthotics serve to alter STJ moments created by these ground reactive forces.
Tissue stress theory of McPoil, Hunt, Fuller, Kirby (1995, 2000, 2002)	-is STJ neutral really the goal? -combination of STJ axis location, rotational equilibrium theory , and kinetic analysis of pathologic stress -Tissue stress occurs when they function beyond their elastic range. -Orthotics keep tissue stress small enough during repetivie loading cycles to prevent plastic deformation and injury to tissue during	-do NOT need to design orthoses to "prevent compensation for foot deformties" or "realign to STJ neutral" -orthoses function to reduce pathological stress on injured tissues -Design orthoses to duplicate internal function of injured tissue so healing can occur: 1) reduce patholotical loading forces on injured structural components

	WB activities	2) optimize gait
		3) prevent other pathologies from occuring
	Fuller- location of center of pressure on plantar foot determines which anatomical structures would most likely be injured	i.e. for plantar fasciitis, the goal is to reduce ground reactive force (GRF): deep heel cup, stiff medial arch, padded topcovers, heel cushion
	McPoil-orthotics mechanically reduce stresses within injured tissues of the body	
Nigg (1999)[130]	orthotics alter the input signals into the plantar foot that cause a change in the "muscle tuning"	

Orthotic definitions[131]

Orthosis	Device to assist, resist, facilitate, stabilze, improve range of motion and function of joints in body
Accomodative orthoses	For rigid/uncompensated deformities, relieves plantar pressure by cushioning. Often made of plastizote, used in DM shoes
	Semi-weight bearing foam foot casting-captures the size and shape of foot
Functional orthoses	The "typical orthotic", controls abnormal biomechanics
Blake inverted orthosis	Puts foot in more supinated position by shifting the ground reactive forces medial to the STJ axis
Kirby medial heel skive	Puts foot in more supinated position by shifting the ground reactive forces medial to the STJ axis
Cobra orthosis	Orthosis designed for high heel shoes where the lateral and center heel are cut away to decrease bulk in shoe
Medial flange	Increase in height of orthosis on medial side just distal to heel and leading up to navicular.
Morton's cutout, reverse Morton's extension (1st ray cutout)	Cutout of a longitudinal band along the first ray, to INCREASE ROM at the first ray to prevent jamming at the 1st MTPJ. Used for hallux limitus/rigidus
Morton's extension	Opposite of Morton's cutout, an addition of material under the 1st MTPJ forming a longitudinal band along the first ray to LIMIT 1st MTPJ ROM
Metatarsal bar	Material added to distal edge of orthosis to transfer force off the metatarsal heads and onto the MT necks and shafts

10 point evalutation of negative cast
- Hallux slightly DF
- 5th digit proximal phalanx parallel to 5th MT shaft
- Thumb impression in sulcus of 4th/5th toes
- Concave 1st MT head impression
- Visible skin lines
- Medial arch slope 2/3
- Accurate forefoot to rearfoot relationship
- Straight lateral border
- Apex of lateral arch under the calcaneocuboid joint
- Rounded heel shape
- Patient and doctor name

Types of gait

Abductory twist	compensation for FF valgus. FF valgus pushed into FF varus by ground, STJ quickly pronates to compensate
Apropulsive gait	pronated foot during propulsion
Antalgic gait	limp
Ataxia/cerebellar gait	WIDE-BASED GAIT, "drunk gait", uncoordinated, jerking, drunk, staggering. seen with MS, tabes dorsalis, DM neuropathy, Fredrich's ataxia
Bouncing gait	early heel off 2/2 equinus

[130] Nigg, Benno M et al "Shoe inserts and orthotics for sport and physical activities." Medicine and science in sports and exercise 31 (1999): S421-S428
[131] http://www.prolaborthotics.com/Education/TermsandDefinitions/tabid/85/Default.aspx

Dyskinetic gait	"writing gait", hyperkinetic, constant variability, motion with considerable effort. Seen with CP, Huntington's chorea, dystonic muscular deformities
Fenestrating gait (shuffling gait)	seen with Parkinson's, slouched over, small short steps
Spastic hemiparesis	drop foot or flexed arm
Scissoring gait (spastic gait)	toe walking and cavus deformity, internal rotation and adduction of entire limb, dragging of distal lateral foot. Seen with CP, spastic diplegia, paraplegia, hemiplegia
Steppage gait	high steps due to SWING PHASE DROP FOOT, weak anterior compartment, limb length. Seen with CMT, polio, Guillain Barre, CVA
Waddling gait	difficulty with balance, pelvic instability, positive Trendelenburg sign. Seen with muscular dystrophies, SMA, congenital dislocated hip
Stomping gait	wide base of gait, legs positioned far apart, stomping on heel
Sensory ataxia	throw feet forward and out, watch ground to walk
Vaulting gait	high step rate, steppage of the side with prosthesis, myotonic dystrophy

Pharmacology

Neuropathy

Drug name	Trade name	Dosage	Max dose	SE
Gabapentin	Neurontin ®	300mg PO tid	3600mg	Sleepiness
Pregabalin	Lyrica ®	50mg PO tid	600mg	
TCA				
Duloxetine	Cymbalta ®	60mg QD		
Capsaicin cream		0.025, 0.075mg		

Local Anesthetics
Ester vs Amide

	Ester	Amide
Name	procaine (novocaine), tetracaine, cocaine, benzocaine	lidocaine, mepivicaine, bupivicaine, etidocaine, prilocaine
Location of detox	BLOOD	LIVER
Length of effect	shorter	longer
Side effects	anaphylaxis	TOXICITY

Toxic dose

Drug	Toxic plain	Toxic epi	Max cc plain	Max cc epi
Lidocaine (Xylocaine ®)	5mg/kg 300 mg	7mg/kg 500mg	30 cc (1%), 15 cc (2%)	50 cc (1%) 25 cc (2%)

Bupivacaine* (Marcaine *, (Exparel *)	2mg/kg 175 mg	3mg/kg 225 mg	35 cc (0.5%), 70 cc (0.25%)	45 cc (0.5%), 90 cc (0.25%)

*Bupivacaine: Cardiac/CNS tox, Not for <12 y.o. due to negative effect on **growth plate**

- Converting % solution into mg: (concentration % x 10) x (# cc's injected)

MOA: bind to voltage gated Na+ channels to block the nociceptive afferent neurons

- Sharp pain, temperature, and touch are carried by **delta fibers**
- With epinephrine:
  - Faster onset, longer duration due to vasoCONSTRICTION, which prevents absorption of anesthetic
    - NO effect in marcaine (lidocaine only)
    - Decreases BLEEDING
- Longer block time in diabetics (poor sensory and motor conduction)
- Anasthetic effect poor in infected area due to low pH. Acidic environment negates effect of anesthetic
- **Exparel:** (liposomal buivicaine)
  - DepoFoam lipid suspension
  - 72 hour anesthetic time
  - Sustained release with decrease in toxicity
  - DO NOT give with other local anesthetic due to risk of toxicity

SE: anxiety, tinnitus, dizziness, restlessness,, allergic reaction, lip numbness, metallic taste, altered level of consciousness
Risk: elderly, children
Systemic toxicity: respiratory failure, seizures, palpitations, cardiac arrest

- Cardiotoxicity-electrophysiologic function, loss of cardiac energy at mitochondria
- TX cardiotoxicity with lipid emulsion to create "lipid pool" to draw out anesthetic from heart
  - Benadryl (diphenhydramine) used as alternative if patient allergic to ester/amide

Reduce SE by: using the lowest concentration and dose necessary, slow injection, repeated aspiration, ultrasound guidance, test dosing, incremental injections (3-5cc), intravascular test dosing

Popliteal block:

Targets sciatic nerve (common peroneal and tibial N)

- better for forefoot cases, less predictable for rear foot cases.
- better coverage for double injection technique distal to sciatic bifurcation
- 14 hour anesthetic coverage
- better success in older age, lower BMI

Double block

- Femoral + sciatic N, good results

Topical Anasthetics

EMLA cream (lidocaine and prilocaine)
Ethyl chloride
Topical lidocaine

General Anesthetics

Malignant hyperthermia:

- Greatest risk during volatile (inhaled) anesthetics,
- CP: respiratory distress, high temperature, high respiratory rate, tachycardia, HTN, electrolyte abnormalities
1. Reverse with DANTROLENE SODIUM

Smoking effects: difficulty with prolonged MAC due to difficulty breathing
Alcohol effects: filter out anasthesia quicker due to high functioning liver that has been forced to detoxify large amounts of alcohol. Give higher doses than normal

General Anesthesia

	time of use	effect	MOA	SE

	time of use	effect	MOA	SE
BZD: #1: midazolam (versed) MC, shortest onset #2: diazepam (valium), #3: lorazepam (ativan),	pre, intra, post operatively Midazolam: no pain with IM/IV (water sol). RETROGRADE AMNESIA	hypnotic, sedative, amnestic, anxiolytic, anticonvulsant, mm relaxant NO ANALGESIA	enhancing inhibitory effects of GABA	resp depression esp midazolam + fentanyl reverse with FLUMAZENIL
propofol (diprivan)	induction, MAC	MC induction hypnotic, sedative, quick return to clear headed state EUPHORIA	GABA and NMDA, direct on spinal cord neurons	egg allergy, resp depression esp + opiates or BZD
etomidate	Induction Good for porphyria ☺	hemodynamic stability CV stability NO ANALGESIA		adrenocortical suppression, N/V
ketamine	Preop, induction, MAC good for peds	CV stimulant to maintain HR, BP, cardiac output, ventilation. sedative, analgesia		vivid dream, out of body, emergence hallucination DISSOCIATIVE ANESTHESIA-cooperate but with analgesia and amnesia SALIVATION
opioids: fentanyl (MC), sufentanil, alfentanil, remifentanil (short)	pre, induction, intra, post operatively	analgesia, hemodynamic stability	synergy + BZD, propofol Fentanyl: 100x potency than morphine	resp depression, hypotension, pruritis, nausea, vomiting, inc ICP, constipation
inhaled: Halogenated: halothane, isoflurane, sevoflurane, desflurane Nonhalogenated: NO	Maintenance	LOC, amnesia, analgesia, depressed consciousness + mm relaxation Halothane: MC ped induction. Only nonvolatile agent (gas at room temp) GOOD: bronchodilator (low resp irritation) NO: good for hx malig hyperthermia rapid induction (low blood gas coefficient)	potentiation of NM blockade, blunting autonomics	(except halothane): Inc bronchial secretion, saliva in smokers→cough, LARYNGOSPASM Enflurane: kidney Halothane: liver, ARRHYTHMIAS 2/2 sensitization to catecholamine NO: BM suppression 2/2 chronic use, HYPOXIA (counteract with 100% O2)
Muscle relaxant: succinyl choline	ET intubation	irreversible mm relaxant	K+ release, so inject SLOWLY	Myalgia CAUTION: myasthenia gravis pts Antidote: neostigmine

	time of use	effect	MOA	SE
Barbiturate (thiopental)	Replaced by BZD, induction	Anxiolytic, sedation		Caution PORPHYRIA (heme dz)
Anticholinergics (belladonna derivative) Glycopyrrolate, scopolamine, atropine	Glycopyrrolate-doesn't cross BBB, less SE ET tube insertion	Reduce resp tract secretions, protect reflex bradycardia, sedative, amnesia		Dry mouth, relaxation of lower esoph sphincter REVERSE with: physostigmine
H2 receptor antag: cimetidine		Prevent aspiration by dec gastric acid		

ASA surgical risk classification

Class	Description
1*	healthy
2*	mild systemic disease (HTN, DM)
3	severe activity-limiting systemic disease (angina, COPD)
4	incapacitating systemic disease constant threat to life
5	moribound patient not expected to survive 24 hours
6	patient declared legally brain dead, awaiting organ harvesting

*40-60% of patients are ASA class 1 or 2

Diuretics

Class	Example	Description	Location	SE
Loop	Furosemide (Lasix)	strong, prevents Na+ reabsorption	ascending loop	increase uric acid or hypoK+.
K+ sparing	Spironolactone (Aldactone)	weak, prevents K+ secretion and Na+ reabsorption	collecting tubules	hyperK+
Thiazide	HCTZ	prevents Na+ reabsorption	distal convoluted tubule	hypoK+

Antidepressant

Class	Example	Description
Tricyclic	Amines, SSRI-Fluoxetine (Prozac), Paroxetine (Paxil), Sertraline (Zoloft)	reduce reuptake of NE or serotonin. may take several weeks to develop.
Antipsychotic	Haloperidol, Clozapine	SE: Parkinsons, tardive dyskinesia

Topical Antibiotics

Drug	Other
Bacitracin (Neosporin ®)	Gram +/-
Bactroban (Mupirocin)	MRSA

Antibiotics

Drug	Coverage	Other
1st gen PCN	Gram + DOC for necrotizing fasciitis, clotridium perfringens	Pen G (IV), Pen V (PO) Dosed in millions of units
2nd gen PCN	Gram +	"PCN-ase resistant": Nafcillin, oxacillin, methicillin
3rd gen PCN	Anaerobes, enterococcus	"AminoPCN": amoxicillin, ampcillin, Augmentin (amoxicillin clavulanate), Unasyn (ampicillin sulbactam)
4th gen PCN	PSEUDOMONAS, gram negative, anaerobes	"Extended-spectrum": Zosyn (pipercillin tazobactam), timentin (ticarcillin clavulanate)
1st gen cephalosporin	Gram + , few gram - PECKS (proteus, e.coli, klebsiella, salmonella, shigella)	cephalexin Keflex ®, cefazolin Ancef ®, **cefadroxil (Duricef®)**
2nd gen cephalosporin	Gram +, **MORE gram -** HEN PECKSS (H. influenza, enterobacter, neisseria, proteus, e.coli, klebsiella, salmonella, shigella)	Cefuroxime (PO), cefotetan (IV)
3rd gen cephalosporin	LESS gram +, **MORE gram -**, PSEUDOMONAS	ceftriaxone Rocephin ®, cefotaxime, ceftazidime, cefexime
4th gen cephalosporin	good gram + and gram - PSEUDOMONAS	cefepime
5th gen cephalosporin	MORE gram +, PSEUDOMONAS, MRSA	ceftaroline
Fluoroquinolones	Gram -, pseudomonas Combine with clindamycin or metronidiazole for DM Levofloxacin: Better staph and strep than cipro	Ciprofloxacin, levofloxacin, moxifloxacin **SE**: asthmatics, tendon rupture, cartilage degeneration in pediatrics, myasthenia gravis
Macrolides	Gram +	Azithromycin, clarithromycin, erythromycin Good for PCN allergy
Aminoglycoside	Gram -, pseudomonas	Gentamycin, tobramycin, amikacin **SE**: Nephrotoxic, ototoxic, monitor peak/trough. Requires O2 for transport into bacteria Use amikacin if resistant to other aminoglycosides

Carbapenem	VRE, Gram +/-, pseudomonas, NO MRSA	Primaxin (cilistatin imipenem), ertapenem (Ivanz) Good for isolated tx of DM foot infection
Sulfonamide (Bactrim)	for UTI, MOA: inhibits bacterial folic acid synthesis	MULTIPLE side effects: **increase effect of warfarin, increase INR/bleed**
Tetracycline (Doxycycline, minocycline, tigecycline)	MRSA, gram +/- but NO pseudomonas good for rickettsia, chlamydia, LYME disease (borrelia burgdorferi), rocky mountain, h. pylori, vibrio vulnificus, mycobacterium pneumoniae	SE: teeth stain, photosensitivity
Lincosamide (Clindamycin)	good for PCN allergy, anaerobes	**SE**: pseudomembranous colitis, cross reaction with macrolid
Chloramphenicol	topical also	**SE**: gray baby syndrome, aplastic anemia (bone marrow suppression)
Metronidazole	good anaerobes	CONTRA pregnancy DOC for pseudomembranous colitis, PO for anaerobes
Rifampin	gram+, legionella, DOC for TB	Never use ALONE **SE**: stains body fluid ORANGE, MRSA, penetrate biofilm
Vancomycin	MRSA	good for implant, covers staph epi PO for pseudomemb colitis and anaerobes, good for PCN allergy
Linezolid (Zyvox) Oxazolidinone	VRE	**SE**: thrombocytopenia, $60 per pill
Synercid (Quinupristin/dalfopristin)	VRE, MRSA	
Daptomycin (cubicin)	MRSA	
Tedizolid (Sivextro)	MRSA	FDA approved for MRSA 6/2014 Less myelosuppression and costs less than linezolid
Ortivancin (orbactiv)	MRSA	FDA approved for MRSA 8/2014 Single dose just as good as BID vancomycin
Dalbavancin (dalvance)	MRSA	FDA approved for MRSA 5/2014 No renal dosing necessary

Pseudomembranous colitis (C. Diff colitis)
ET: normal gut flora gets wiped out by strong antibiotic. Normal gut flora replaced by clostridium difficile. C.diff releases toxins that cause bloating, diarrhea, abdominal pain.
RF: broad spectrum ABx: clindamycin, fluoroquinolones, cephalosporins, carbapenems
TX: metronidazole, PO Vanco, STOOL TRANSPLANT

Surgical prophylactic Antibiotics:
- Give within 1 hour of incision
- For dirty wounds, valvular heart dz, surgery time >2 hours, implants, blood transfusion: give Ancef, if PCN allergy: vancomycin

Dosages of commonly used Antibiotics

Abx	Route	Dose

PCN G	IV	12-24 million units QD
Keflex ® (cephalexin)	PO	500mg Q6 x 7-10 days
Clindamycin	IV/PO	300mg PO Q8 600mg IV Q8
Ancef ® (cefazolin)	IV	1g IV per 70kg Q8 x 3
Vancomycin	IV/PO	**1g IV Q12 slow infusion*** 125mg PO Q6 *some sources may suggest trough of 15-20, but for most pts with SSTI who have normal renal function, not obese, 1g Q12 is adequate and trough monitoring not required[132]
Bactrim ® Septra ® (TMP/SMX)	PO	80 TMP/400 SMX PO BID DS: 160/400
Ciprofloxacin	IV/PO	250-750mg PO BID 200-400mg IV BID
Zyvox ® (linezolid)	PO	600mg PO BID
Zyvox ® (linezolid)	IV	600mg IV Q12
Amoxicillin	PO	250-500mg TID
Unasyn	IV	3g IV Q6 1.5g IV Q6 for renal
Erythromycin	PO	250-500mg Q6
Augmentin	PO	500/125mg TID
Zosyn	IV	3.375g IV Q4-6 4.5g IVQ8
Flagyl (metronidazole)	PO	500mg PO Q8
Ertapenem (Ivanz ®)	IV/IM	1g QD

Peaks and trough
Peak: measure 30 minutes after 3rd dose
Trough: measure 30 minutes before 4th dose
Vanco
- peak: 15-30 mg/ml
- trough: <10 mg/ml
Gentamycin
- peak: 5-10 mg/ml
- trough: <2 mg/ml

Schedule drugs

Schedule	Definition

[132] Stevens, Dennis L., et al. "Practice guidelines for the diagnosis and management of skin and soft tissue infections: 2014 update by the Infectious Diseases Society of America." Clinical Infectious Diseases 59.2 (2014): e10-e52.

1	No therapeutic use (heroin)
2	Non-refillable, cannot call in (hydrocodone)
3	Refillable 5x in 6 months (Tylenol #3)
4	Low abuse potential
5	OTC

Opioid (Narcotics)

MOA: bind to Mu, Delta, Kappa receptors

SE: Constipation --> toxic megacolon, hypotension, respiratory depression, nausea, urinary retention, drowsiness, opioid induced hyperalgesia (OIH), pruritis, miosis, euphoria
- Suppressed cough reflex in low dose
- CONTRAINDICATED in head trauma due to increase in ICP

Drug	Dose	Other
Norco ® (hydrocodone & acetaminophen)	5/325 or 10/325 Q6 PRN	Toxic dose: limited by acetaminophen: max 4000mg/day
Vicodin ® (hydrocodone & acetaminophen)	5/300 or 5/500 Q6 PRN	
Percocet ® (oxycodone & acetaminophen)	5/325 Q6 PRN	
Fentanyl patch (Sublimaze ®)	2.5-10mg	Synthetic opioid
MS (morphine sulfate) Contin	30mg PO BID 2mg IV Q4	
Dilaudid ® (hydromorphone)	2mg PO Q6 PRN 2mg IM	Good for renal failure patients
Tylenol #3 ® (codeine & acetaminophen)	30/300 PO Q6	Used for cough
Oxycontin ® (oxycodone)		

Pain medication (opioid allergy)

Drug	MOA	Toxic dose
Tramadol (Ultram ®)	**Mu opioid antagonist + SNRI** (serotonin/NE re-uptake inhibition)	Max 4000mg/day
Toradol (Ketorolac)	NSAID (COX inhibition)	
Acetaminophen (Tylenol ®), paracetamol, APAP	COX inhibition	4000mg/day
Methocarbamol (Robaxisal)		

NSAIDS

MOA: COX inhibition to prevent production of prostaglandins

USE: anti-inflammatory, antipyretic, analgesic

SE: Delayed bone healing, increased bleeding (CONTRA in GI ulcer, take with food to decrease GI irritation), asthmatic attack (COX inhibition increases leukotriene production, a bronchoconstrictor), nausea, interstitial nephritis

Class	Drug	Dose	Other
Salicyclate	Aspirin (Bayer ®)	325-1g PO Q4-6	4000mg/day (IRREVERSIBLE). DOC for RA Increase bleeding time *causes Reye's syndrome in children with viral illness DO NOT use for: gout (inhibit uric acid excretion), asthmatic, coumadin
Propionic acid derivative	Ibuprofen (Advil ®, Motrin ®)	300-800mg PO Q4-6	Max dose: 2400mg/day
Propionic acid derivative	Naproxen (Aleve ®)	250-500mg PO BID	
Acetic acid derivative	Indomethacin		used to treat gout
COX-2 inhbitor	Celecoxib		COX 2 inhibitor, good for those with stomach problems, taking anticoagulants, CONTRA in sulfa allergy
COX-2 inhbitor	Nabumetone (Relafen®)		for arthritis
Acetic acid derivative	Ketorolac (Toradol ®)	30mg IV Q6 10mg PO Q6 PRN	No more than 5 days due to nephrotoxicity
Acetic acid derivative	Diclofenac (Arthrotec ®)	75mg PO or TOPICAL	Arthrotec ® coated with misoprostol to dec gastritis
Arylalkanoic acid	Sulindac		for OA, low GI irritation
Oxicam derivative	Piroxicam (Feldene ®)		QD dosing
anti-malarial	Hydrochloroquine (Plaquenil)		tx RA, malaria, SLE
Oxicam derivative	Meloxicam (Mobic)		for OA
COX and LOX	licofeldone, tepoxalin		

Antidotes

Drug	Antidote
anticholinesterase	atropine (ACLS)
Benzodiazepine	Flumazenil
Digoxin	digoxin immune antibody
methanol	ethanol
iron	deferoxamine (DMSA)

lead	succimer
methotrexate	leucovorin calcium (folinic acid)
TCA	physostigmine
ASA	NaHCO3
opioid	naloxone (narcan)

Steroid injections

	Acetate	Phosphatate
Trade name	Triamcinolone (Kenalog)	Dexamethasone (Decadron)
Water solubility	Non-water soluble (white precipitate)	Water soluble
Injection location	Muscle	Joint
Length	long acting	short acting

- **Betamethasone** can be both acetate or phosphatate
- 1:1:1:0.75:0.75 lidocaine, bupivacaine, kenalog, dexamethasone
- SE of steroids:
    - Topical: striae, HYPERpigmentation, atrophy, rosacea (facial redness), peri-orbital dermatitis
    - Injection: skin necrosis, HYPOpigmentation, steroid flare (INTENSE PAIN, will get better), skin/fat atrophy, hypersensitivity, muscle wasting
    - Oral: adrenal suppression, impaired wound healing, Cushing's syndrome, hyperglycemia
        - ☐ NEED TO WEAN OFF to prevent Addison's like symptom due to negative feedback mechanism of oral steroids

Cushings vs Addison's syndrome

	Cushings	Addisons
Cortisol	HIGH	LOW
Symptoms	HYPOpigmentation, buffalo hump, moon facies, thinning of arms and legs	HYPERpigmentation, hypoglycemia, weight loss, muscle weakness
Na+ and blood pressure	Increased	Decreased
K+	Decreased	increased
Etiology	Hypersecretion of ACTH from pituitary adenoma, XS cortisol	Abrupt cessation of steroid therapy

Topical steroid

Drug	Intensity
1% hydrocortisone	Mild
Triamcinolone	Moderate
Betamethasone, clobetasol	Potent

DM medication

Drug	Class	Details

Drug	Class	Details
metformin (glucophage)	Biguanide	first line tx contraindicated in imparied renal, hepatic function no risk for hypoglycemia SE: GI, bloating, N/V/D **BBW: LACTIC ACIDOSIS**
Glyburide, glipizide	sulfonylurea	weight gain, hypoglycemia
Glitazone	TZD	8-12 weeks for effect SE: fluid retention
Meglitinide		increases insulin secretion

Antiemetics

Drug	Trade name
Odansetron	Zofran
Metaclopramide	Reglan
Olanzapine	Zyprexa
Promethazine	Phenergan
Compazine	Prochlorperazine

Procedures

Nail matrixectomy
Nerve block
- 3 ccs of lidocaine per toe
- Drawing needle
- Injection needle
- Syringe
- Alcohol pads

Avulsion
- Betadine
- Tourniquet—wrap distally —> proximally
- Free with spatula
1. English anvil
- Curved hemostat—rotate towards center of nail
- Phenol-30 seconds, rotating towards the center of the nail
- Neutralizing solution-alcohol/saline

Dressing
- Spread antibiotics on the toe
- Use the 4x4 to wrap around toe once, wrap with the long thin gauze
- Wrap with coban

Follow up
- 2 weeks

Bier block
- Exsanguinate limb
- Tourniquet
  - Inject anesthetic into veins, which are close to nerve, will diffuse there
  6. Release tourniquet to stop nerve block

AO Screw insertion: (Scripps found better results with over drilling first)
- <u>Under drill</u>-DISTAL core diameter, engages distal cortex, allows retrograde compression
- <u>Over drill</u>-PROXIMAL thread diameter prevent retrograde compression
- <u>Countersink</u>-enables screw head flush with bone
- <u>Measure</u>
- <u>Tap</u>-creates thread lines (most screws are now are self-tapping)
- <u>Insert</u>

AO screw insertion: placing 2 screws:
First screw: perpendicular to both cortices
Second/third screw: perpendicular to fracture at an angle to bisect the angle between the fracture and cortical surface

Effect of corticosteroids on bone healing
- Promote apoptosis of osteoblast and osteocytes —> osteonecrosis
- Extend lifespan of osteoclasts
- Increase excretion of Ca2+

Order of ossification of bones in foot
Calcaneus, talus cuboid, lateral cuneiform, medial cuneiform, intermediate cuneiform, navicular, sesamoid
- birth: **cuboid,** talus, calcaneus, MT, phalanges,
- 1 year: **lateral cuneiform**, cuboid, talus, calcaneus, MT, phalanges,
- 2 year: **medial cuneiform**, lateral cuneiform, cuboid, talus, calcaneus, MT, phalanges
- 3 year: **2nd cuneiform**, medial cuneiform, lateral cuneiform, cuboid, talus, calcaneus, MT, phalanges
- 4th year: **navicular**, 2nd cuneiform, medial cuneiform, lateral cuneiform, cuboid, talus, calcaneus, MT, phalanges

Ossified at birth:
Calcaneus, talus, cuboid, MT shaft, phalanges

Preparing all surgery
- Roll of padding under tourniquet
- Steri drape 1000 (1010 if using ankle tourniquet)
- Drawing local anaesthesia: draw with the smaller gauge, inject with the bigger gauge (bigger gauge = smaller diameter)

Austin bunionectomy
- Mayo block
- Dorsomedial incision
  - dissection: watch out for tendon medial to EHL: extensor hallucis capsularis (freshman nerve), found in 88%, originates from EHL tendon, inserts into 1st MTPJ capsule
- Lateral release:
  - Adductor hallucis
  - Fibular sesamoid ligament
  - FHB tenotomy
  - Fibular sesamoidectomy
- Capsulotomy to expose MT head
  - can consider repair of medial collateral ligament (Swedish)
- Free MT head
- Determine how much medial MT to excise (Silver) using fluoroscopy
- Excise using saw
- Suture capsule (Vicryl)
- Suture skin-Vicryl for subcut, then nylon superficially to tighten
Chevron osteotomy

- o   Use a 0.045 inch k wire as axis guide (axis guide just below midpoint of MT head)
- Plantar arm first
- K wire directed perpendicular to MT shaft = maintain length
  - Directed more anteriorly: lengthen
  - Directed more posteriorly: shorten
- Use a 0.045 k wire to maintain translocation while focusing on permanent fixation
- 0.062 inch k wire:
- perpendicular to plantar of osteotomy in lateral view, pointing to cristae
- remove k wire
- underdrill distal
- overdrill proximal
- countersink
- depth gauge
- insert screw
- remove temporary fixation

Long dorsal arm-corrects larger IM angles
- Dorsal arm first
- Use 2 screws, perpendicular to dorsal arm
  - Countersink distal screw > proximal screw

Complications:
- AVN, recurrence, transfer metatarsalgia, hallux varus, nonunion, malunion

1st MPJ fusion
- remove all osteophytes
- ream 1st MT head and base of proximal phalanx
- secure with screws and plate
- prep point with subchondral drilling, secure with screws, lag only one of them
- union in 8-12 weeks

1st MPJ hemi-implant (osteomed)
- remove osteophytes off 1st MT head
- measure size of base of proximal phalanx with sizer
- make hole for implant to be inserted in
- medial capsulorraphy by cutting around kelly forcep

Lapidus bunionectomy
- extensile medial incision from proximal phalanx to midfoot
- make sure to avoid medial marginal vein (great saph)
- lateral release of sesamoid collateral ligament, lateral capsule,
- capsulotomy of 1st MCJ
  - planing of the 1st MCJ using saw, removing cartilage and not subchondral bone
  - position 1st ray in rectus position
  - K wire to temporary fixate
  - Screw #1 (most important, "home-run screw", 3.5 or 4.0) from **dorsal (1st MT base)** —> **plantar medial (medial cuneiform)**:
    - important to properly countersink 1st MT shaft to create adequate notch through dorsal cortex for screw head to enter
    - lag technique
    - almost parallel to ground, grab as much cortex as possible
  - Screw #2 at 1st MT plantar to first screw, through 2nd, even 3rd MT
- Screw #3 from **dorsal (medial cuneiform)** —> **plantar medial (1st MT base)**
- Screws cross **DISTAL** to MCJ (in 1st MT base)
- **Shear-strain-relieved bone graft**:
  - trough created at TMTJ and packed with cancellous autograft
  - eliminates shear stress
- To prevent shortening of 1st ray:
  - bone graft

- PF 1st ray

Lisfranc arthrodesis
- Incision in first interspace and over 4th MT. At least 4cm apart
- Caution superficial peroneal N, deep perineal N, dorsalis pedis (1cm distal to 1st TMTJ)
- Prep joints
- Reduction forceps between 2nd MT and medial cuneiform
  - **Screw #1**: K-wire through 1st TMTJ, insert 3.5 or 4.0 screw
  - **Screw #2**: 2nd MT base through medial cuneiform

TN fusion
- incision between med mal and TA from ankle to NCJ
- avoid medial marginal vein (great saph.)
- baby laminar spreader to open joint
- osteotome to remove subchondral bone
- fenestrate bone with 0.062 K wire

Triple arthrodesis
- ⬚ want to ensure plantigrade foot
- ⬚ TN fusion gives 92% fusion to STJ[133]
- ⬚ don't even really need to fuse CC joint
- start with STJ with lateral incision
- prep the joint with fish scaling then subchondral drilling
- 2x 6.5 1/4 threaded cannulated screws from calcaneus horizontally, one through anterior facet, one through posterior facet. Do not need to countersink.
- then fuse TNJ

Triple Arthrodesis

30 weeks for fusion
- medial incision exposing STJ and TNJ
  - o caution great saphenous vein
- T-incision for TNJ
  - o caution PTT
- resect talar head cartilage
- lateral incision exposing STJ and CCJ
  - o caution EDB muscle belly, communicating branch of sural N to intermediate dorsal cutaneous nerve, peroneus tertius tendon
- deep fascia separation and reflection of EDB
  - o caution venous plexus
- inverted L incision over CCJ
  - o remove hoke's tonsil
  - fish scale pattern over calcaneus in CCJ
  - contour resection of cartilage over STJ
  - Steinmann pins to temporary fixate
  - 6.5mm or 7.0mm cannulated screws
  - STJ screw: dorsomedial talar neck —> posterolateral calcaneus
  - TNJ screw: distal-inferomedial navicular—> middle of talar dome
  - CCJ screw: distal dorsolateral cuboid —> under sustentaculum tali
- insert closed-suction drain

Hammertoe surgery
- Dorsal elliptical incision, remove skin
- Cut extensor tendons to expose PIPJ
- Pull aside vv and cauterize if necessary
- Cut collateral ligaments (can use **beaver blade**)
- Use a bone shear to cut head of proximal phalanx (can smooth out using **rongeur**)

---

[133] Astion, Donna J., et al. "Motion of the Hindfoot after Simulated Arthrodesis*." The Journal of Bone & Joint Surgery 79.2 (1997): 241-6.

- Insert k-wire down the base of the middle phalanx distally out the toe, leaving a tip
- Drive the wire back down through the proximal phalanx
- Cut k wire and bend, placing a bead at the tip
- Splint the toe:
    - MTPJ: slightly PF
    - PIPJ: straight
    - DIPJ: straight
- Suture extensor tendon (Vicryl)
- Suture skin (nylon)
- *Make sure toe does not remain white after releasing tourniquet
- Swelling may not go away for 6-12 months (or never go away) because of small lymphatics in the toe
- K-wire removal in 3 weeks
- Complications
    - Lateral deviation of hammertoe—treat with Budin splint
    - Postop swelling/pain
    - Arthroplasty-recurrent hammertoe. A good idea to fuse the 2nd PIPJ
    - Hemosiderin deposit
        - Hematoma-a damage vessel leading to severe edema, erythema, serosanguineous drainage, induration, pain on palpation

TMA
- Palpate and approximate location of each MT head
- If amputation done >1 year ago, can make new incision separate from original one
- Visualize MT head and bone spicule
- Excise bone spicule using **osteotome** and hammer
- Smooth out tip of bone using osteotome
- Save bone spicule for lab testing
- Vicryl subcut then secure with nylon
- Debride ulcer generously, even to point of bleeding
- Dress the wound
- **PEARLS**: GENTLE with soft tissue, do not pinch down forceps but use only to fold back tissue. Do not need to bevel bone, can just do vertical cut. Simple interrupted with 3.0 nylon has less constriction of skin than horizontal mattress.

Tibial Sesamoidectomy
- Anatomy:
    - Sesamoid apparatus: plantar plate, intersesamoid ligament, tibial/fibular sesamoid ligaments (medial/lateral sesamoid MT ligament), phalangeal sesamoidal ligaments (distal/plantar sesamoid ligaments)
- Mayo block (1st ray block)
    - Medial dorsal cutaneous nerve, saphenous nerve, medial terminal branch of deep peroneal nerve, first common and proper plantar digital nerve
        - Dorsum of foot and redirect medially
        - Plantar medial of foot, under first MT
        - First interspace
        - Medial hallux
- Medial incision along hallux, (dot on dorsal and plantar MT, find the middle), avoiding the medial dorsal cutaneous nerve dorsally, medial plantar nerve plantarly. (Hiss approach)
    - Dorsomedial approach (Mcbride) between extensor tendon
    - Prox at neck of MT
- Expose the capsule
- Incise the capsule dorsomedially to the tibial sesamoid
    - Linear incision superior to abductor hallucis
- Free the tendon attachment of the abductor hallucis, FHB, tibial sesamoid ligament, intersesamoid ligament, and "shell" out the sesamoid
- Close the capsule with absorbable suture (Vicryl)
- Complications:
    - Arthritic joints results in calcified ligaments = difficult to release
- Use a osteotome to release

- o Bipartite sesamoids may result in sesamoid coming out in smaller and multiple pieces
    - ▢ Use a K-wire as joystick to be able to manipulate the sesamoid
- o FHL runs plantarly under the intersesamoid ligament. It can be nicked or cut.
- Pearls:
    - o Make sure to leave enough soft tissue on the sesamoid so that you can grasp the sesamoid and manipulate it to expose the other ligaments
        - o Use the K wire earlier to take out sesamoid in one piece instead of a rongeur, which breaks the sesamoid into smaller pieces
    - Indications:
        - o Recurrent ulcer
        - Fracture
        - OM
        - Arthritis
    - Bunions w/ arthritis (hallux limitus/rigidus)
        - **Sesamoiditis**
    - **Bipartite sesamoidectomy**

Soft tissue Cavus foot reconstruction (Gastroc recession, plantar fasciotomy, peroneus longus release)
- Tourniquet at 300 mmHg
    - **Numb all 3 locations with 20 cc Marcaine**
- Cast in a bivalve below the knee cast converted into a posterior splint.
    - D/C with Vicodin 5/500 mg PO Q4 PRN
1) Gastrocnemius recession—endoscopic or open
2) Plantar fasciotomy—(posterior tibial nerve block), horizontal incision at distal aspect of heel where fatty tissue remains, between medial and lateral margins of central band. Cut the fascia with toes in DF (fascia feels like celery, deep to it is the FDB). Lavage with saline. Close with horizontal mattress. Ambulate the next day.
    a. Endoscopic plantar fasciotomy-less pain, earlier return to activity
3) Peroneus longus release—2cm incision on lateral aspect right above peroneal tendons, just posterior to the fibula, 6cm proximal to ankle joint. Dissect through tendon sheath. Locate the peroneus longus superficial to the peroneus brevis. Tug on tendons to double check which tendons are which. Make sure all fibers of tendon are together, and cut with scissors. Remove a small piece of tendon. Lavage the area with saline. Suture tendon sheath together with Vicryl, close with horizontal mattress.

Ankle ORIF, ankle fracture
- lateral incision
    - anterolateral incision: CAUTION: superficial peroneal
- dissect with peroneus tertius anteriorly, PB/PL posteriorly
- align fracture in anatomic position, hold with lobster claw forcep or K-wire, C-arm for alignment
    - **interfrag screw** perpendicular to fracture in lag technique
        - for a 3.5 screw, 2.5 underdrill, 3.5 overdrill, countersink, measure, screw
- **1/3 tubular neutralization plate, 5-8 holes** over fracture, bent to fit shape of fibula, with at least 4 cortices on each side (except on proximal side, which has danger of entering the joint space)
    - Posterior placement greater stability
    - 2x 4.0 **cancellous screws** distal to fracture line
        - drill using 2.5 drill bit (fluoro to help gauge how deep you are)
        - aim in oblique fashion to grab as much cancellous bone as possible, careful not to disrupt joint space
    - 2x 3.5 **cortical screws** proximal to fracture line
        - 2.5 drill bit
        - aim perpendicular to bone
- interfrag screw in lag fashion to secure butterfly fragments

Talar En-block
Medial OCD
- medial incision
- oblique tibial osteotomy
- hinge at deltoid exposing medial talus
- remove piece of talus, match to allograft

- insert talus with 2x 2.0 cannulated headless screw
- fixate tibia with 2 x parallel 6.5 cannulated headless screws
o   put in AO splint

Tibial osteotomy with modified Chrisman Snook
o   for chronic ankle instability secondary to tibial varum component
o   opening tibial wedge ostetomy with medial approach, using deltoid ligament as hinge
o   use a PL allograft to anchor at calcaneus, route through fibula, anchor at talus, and then anchor at sinus tarsi

Peroneal stop procedure (Peroneus longus-brevis tenodesis)
o   dissect to visualize peroneal synovial sheath, first see peroneus longus (peroneus brevis deep)
o   remove peroneal tubercle if enlarged
  o   prep tendon by grazing it with #15 blade
  o   suture tendons together with fiber wire

Endoscopic gastrocnemius recession
- Increases ankle DF by 15 degrees

Indications
- Diabetic patients with peripheral neuropathy and loss of sural nerve function (Trevino FAI 2005[134])

Contraindications
- Excess adipose tissue—should do open GR (Roukis[135])
- PAD

Caution
- Sural nerve injury
1. Great saphenous vein injury

- Patient in supine position
- Sterile thigh/high calf tourniquet @ 300mmHg
- (Tibial nerve (popliteal block)—5-7 cm proximal to skin crease, 0.5-1cm lateral to midline of popliteal fossa)
- Posteromedial incision at the border of the gastroc tendon, ~10cm proximal to ankle, slightly posterior to the medial malleolus, through the crural fascia.
- DF the ankle to view gastroc borders
- Insert fascial elevator to protect subcut tissue, insert camera to visualize gastroc aponeurosis dorsally. DF/PF foot to see the tendon gliding.
- Insert blade and make one straight cut, DF ankle as you cut.
  o   (Residual medial and lateral fibers can be cut with Metzenbaum scissors)
- Check ankle DF to see if it has increased
- Lavage the area with saline
- Close area with 3-0 Vicryl, 4-0 nylon.
- Dress wound with adaptic and gauze. Splint using the posterior shell of a cast.
  o   Cast the patient normally
  o   Make "L cuts" on either side of the cast, and pull the anterior piece off, throw away.

Hoke Tendoachilles lengthening (TAL)
- Percutaneous incisions medial, lateral and medial 3cm apart from each other
- First incision 2cm proximal to insertion of Achilles
- Close incision sites with suture
- Posterior splint
  1. SE: increased heel pressure —> ulceration

Transmetatarsal amputation (TMA)
- Perform with TAL and posterior splint
- Disarticulate MTPJ 1-5 with scalpel

---

[134] Trevino, Saul, Mark Gibbs, and Vinod Panchbhavi. "Evaluation of results of endoscopic gastrocnemius recession." *Foot & ankle international* 26.5 (2005): 359-364.

[135] Roukis, Thomas S., and Monica H. Schweinberger. "Complications associated with uni-portal endoscopic gastrocnemius recession in a diabetic patient population: an observational case series." *The journal of Foot and Ankle Surgery* 49.1 (2010): 68-70.

- Key elevator to free up tissue at MT heads
    - Sagittal saw to cut MT heads, bevel the edges of the bone
        1. Maintain MT parabola
    - Scalpel to remove MT heads by hugging the bone
    - Pull and cut the extensor tendons/collateral ligaments/remaining tissue
    - 300mL saline lavage
    - Close flap with horizontal mattress
    - NWB

COMPLICATION
    - Equinovarus—loss of long extensors/flexors, which are the stabilizers of the foot
        o also lose everting force of PB
        o Secure with posterior splint

Charcot recon
- ⬚ IM bolt
- 1st MT head to talar body
- posterior plantar calcaneus to talar body

Tendon transfer
    - Only for flexible/semi rigid deformities
    - Myotendinous junction is the weakest part of tendon
    - Types of tendon
        o Endotenon —> epitenon —> paratenon
        o Mesotenon-loose, non-friction, vascular attachments
        o Vincula-partial mesotenon
        o Plica-double fold of tendon at proximal and distal tendon sheath to prevent tears

Tendon anchors
    - Expandable-cortical penetration, more difficult to remove
        o barbed anchors, winged anchors
    - Screw type-cancellous penetration, less anchoring strength
    - Materials: metallic, non metallic (PEEK), resorbable (PLLA, PLDLA)

Wound vac
    o Clean entire foot and wound with betadine, rinse with saline
    o Debride wound until bleed, measure
    o Tincture of benzoin around wound for adhesive
    o (Insert soaked white sponge cut to fit snugly in wound)
    o Lay a big black sponge over white sponge
    - Cover with adhesive, using as many pieces as desired
        o Cut dime shape out of the adhesive of each ulcer
- Use a black sponge to build a bridge between two separate ulcers
    - Lay suction over black sponge with tube proximally

Total contact cast (TCC) application
    o Interdigital cushioning
    o Stockingette 3 fingers under fibular head
    o Pad to tibial crest to dorsum of foot, cut to fit forefoot piece, medial and lateral malleoli
    o Prone position, 90 degrees
    o Plaster
    o Fiberglass
    o Posterior splint of fiberglass
    o Heel pad made from folds of fiberglass

AFO (ankle foot orthoses)
    - Prevent ankle PF
    - Richie brace-restricts foot to only sagittal motion of ankle
        - can restrict amount of ankle DF/PF
    - Arizona brace (gauntlet AFO)

7. UCBL (University of California Biomechanics/Berkeley Lab)
   - deep heel cup
   o for flexible deformity

Casting/splinting

- Foot at 90 degrees!!

Plaster	Fiberglass
Easier to mold	Difficult to mold
Not water resistant	Better imaging
Generates more heat	Generates less heat
Better for fracture reduction	Lightweight, stronger

-

AO splint plaster:
   o Stockingette
   o Webril
   o Sugar tong: slab of 5 along med/lateral mall
   o Posterior splint: slab of 10 along foot and posterior calf
   a. Webril
   o ACE

Jones' splint/Jones' compression dressing
   o WAWA (webril ACE, webril ACE)
   o can add posterior splint if desired or put in CAM boot
   o for ankle reduction, Lisfranc

Low-dye taping
- 2 x 1" Heel lock: proximal to base of 1st to base of 5th
   o Hold foot in supinated position during taping
- 3-4 x 2" Plantar rest straps: anterior heel to metatarsal bases
   - (optional) 1" dorsal strap

Hardware

Hardware

Plate	Biomechanical Function
Buttress plate	**MOA**: A "wall" that acts as bridge between larger fragments with intervening small fragments leaning against the plate. Prevent shearing/bending forces Usually for peri/intra-articular fractures at the end of long bone (distal tibia/pilon fracture) Use on tension (convex) side of injury, contoured, serve as cortex. T/L/cloverleaf/spoon design

Plate	Biomechanical Function
Neutralization (protection) plate	Applied to fractures already reduced/compressed with **lag screw** placed outside of plate. Redistribution of force through plate + interfrag compression. <u>Protects interfrag screw fixation from torsional forces.</u> All **concentric** screws
Anti-glide	**A neutralization plate placed on posterior fibula.** Dynamic compression, for **posterior** Weber B fibular fracture. **Posterior plate** wedges fragment in place where axial load provides compressive force. Useful for osteoporosis. Can be performed with 1/3 tubular plate
Compression plate (static, dynamic)	**Static:** compression at fracture. Eccentric drilling of first 2 screws. The rest of the screws can be inserted concentrically. **Dynamic:** compression at fracture AND when implant subjected to physiological load. Follows concept of <u>tension band fixation-place plate on side of TENSION (convex side), NOT compression side</u> Used when lag screw fixation not enough. applies stress parallel to plate with 3 **MOA:** over-bend plate, tension device, screw insertion geometry
Bridging plate	"Neutralization plate without interfrag screw" maintain length and alignment of severely comminuted fractures. **Wave plate:** for areas of delayed healing, contoured away from (comminuted/pseudoarthrosis) to allow bone graft and better ingrowth of vessels
Hook plate	for small/comminuted medial malleolar fragments. could be fashioned from 1/3 tubular plate
Limited contact plate	grooves on the underside of the plate that limit periosteal contact
Tension band	2 parallel K-wires reverses tension (convex side) and turns it into compression. Good for avulsion fracture, malleoli, small fragment, comminuted fracture.
Stainless steel wire	for IPJ fusion Pro: osteoporotic bone, splintage Con: no compression, tendon irritation

Plate	Shape/Design
Axial/dynamic compression plate i.e. 1/3 tubular plate	the 1/3 refers to 1/3 the circumference of the cylinder Can have thick, oval, sloped holes Pre-bend plate away from bone cortex. Tubular design-edges dig into periosteum **1) neutralization mode**-centered **2) compression mode**-1mm "eccentricly" away from fracture line (eyes "looking out" for your patient) **3) buttress mode**-1mm "eccentricly" towards fracture line
Limited contact-dynamic compression (LCDC)	underside of plate contoured for compression in different directions. Better distribution of stress to plate, less hardware failure
Locking plate	Evenly distributes force across ENTIRE screw. Screw and plate function as ONE unit instead of separate units. Multiple screws can be added w/o losing reduction In non-locking screw, shear force is concentrated at HEAD of screw. Unless plate is molded to bone, compression by screw can induce loss of reduction

Plate	Shape/Design
Reconstruction plate	notches allow for easier bending

External fixation
- **Monolateral**-length and stability
- **Circular (Ilizarov)**-smooth, non-threaded wires under tension provide stability
  - FWB s/p surgery to improve rehab, minimizing postoperative osteoporosis

Type of Screw	Function
Cortical screw	large core diameter = increased strength
Shaft screw	partially threaded, shaft diameter = external thread diameter. For interfrag compression
Cancellous screw	when used as lag, entire length of thread should be in fracture fragment
Malleolar screw	partially threaded self cutting cortical screw
Herbert screw	Headless screw proximal and distal threads separated by smooth shaft. Allows for insertion through **cartilage**. leading threads have greater pitch. some compression
Lag screw	**Right angle to fracture**-MAX interfrag compression, but MIN axial stability **Right angle to long axis of bone**-MAX axial stability, can cause dislocation of fragments as it is tightened —>Have one screw (central screw) perpendicular to the long axis of bone and the rest perpendicular to fracture

Screws/fixation

	Cancellous	Cortical
Threads	Deep and widely spaced	Shallow and closely spaced
Self tapping*	Yes	No
Use	As lag screws for metaphyseal fractures	**1st MT** Plate fixation through both cortices, blunt tip protrude few mm into soft tissue

*Self-tapping: cut own thread pattern-not recommended to use as lag screw (may not purchase under drill and you will never know it, since it cut its own thread path)

Drill bit sizes

Mini frag (overdrill → underdrill)	Small frag (2.5 underdrill)	Large frag (3.2 underdrill)
1.5—>1.1	3.5	4.5
2.0—>1.5	4.0	6.5
2.7—>2.0		

Perioperative

PMHx

Condition	Details
HTN	2+ BP readings >140/90. delay surgery if BP> 200/120 Labs: BUN, EKG, creatinine continue medication
CAD, angina, MI	postpone surgery after MI for 6wks-6mo maintain HR <70bpm continue beta blockers and statins Anticoagulants-D/C 3-6 days prior to surgery, resume 24 hours postop. If not possible, d/c Coumadin 3 days prior to surgery, start heparin drip. NSAIDs (Advil, naproxen): D/C 1 week
Valvular disease, murmur	no prophylaxis indicated
Pacemakers, AICD	keep electrocautery to minimum
Pulmonary disease	Pulse ox to monitor O2 sat continue medications
DM	blood glucose control, convert to ISS perioperatively EKG, CBC, BMP frequent blood glucose checks **NIDDM day of surgery**: hold oral hypoglcemics, metformin **IDDM day of surgery**: 1/2-1/3 daily dose of intermediate insulin if BS > 300
OSA, obesity	OSA-increased sensitivity to opiates
Hematologic disease	preoperative CBC **Sickle cell**-NO LE tourniquet due to inc acidosis, hypoxia, venous stasis. Risk hypoxia, low cardiac output, unstable BP
Geriactric	increased sensitivity to BZD
Pediatric	
Malignant hyperthermia	ET: rare autosomal dominant disorder, reaction to halogenated anesthesia (halothane) + succinylcholine leading to reduced re-uptake of Ca2+ by sarcoplasmic reticulum CP: fasciculation, increased muscle tone, clenched jaw, rigidity, inc O2 consumption, inc CO2 production, tachycardia, hyperthermia, rhabdomyolysis TX: dantrolene sodium, cool with iced IV Saline
Thyroid storm	fever, dehydration, tachycardia, weakness,

- Labs-NEITHER MEDICALLY APPROPRIATE NOR HELPFUL

- o Refer to anasthesiologist
- o CBC, Chem 7, coag panel, vitals, HbA1C, preop antibiotics, pregnancy, UA, glucose POC
  - ▪ Chem 7 = Chem 6 + creatinine
  - ▪ Coag panel-if on Coumadin

Lab Values Summary

	Description	Normal
WBC	**Leukocytosis**: bacterial infection, inflammatory process, tissue necrosis, stress **Leukopenia**: overwhelming infection, BM suppression, chemotherapy	4-12
Hgb		14-18 male 12-16 female
ESR	**Westergren method**: distance erythrocytes fall in a column of anticoagulated blood due to gravity **Low ESR**: NORMALLY, negatively charged erythrocytes repel each other decreasing Rouleaux formation **High ESR**: infection releases fibrinogen, decreasing the negatively charged erythrocytes, decreasing their repelling forces. Increase in Rouleaux formation __Chronic__ measure for inflammation **ESR unaffected by DM** **ESR not elevated in chronic OM, recent antibiotic treatment**	<20 normal 20-60 moderate **>80 severe** (estimate: male: age/2 female: age/2 + 10)
CRP	$$, liver protein found only during inflammation __Acute__ measure for inflammation	<1 normal
PT/PTT	PT: increased by vitamin K deficiency, coumadin PTT: increased by hemophilia, von willebrand, DIC	
INR		3-4 normal
Albumin	Decreased with inflammation and malnutrition Transport drugs, easy drug toxicity if albumin low	>3.5 normal 3-3.5 mild 2.5-3 moderate <2.5 severe
BUN	Increased in renal failure Decreased in liver failure	5-25
Creatinine		0.6-1.2mg/dL
K+	HypoK+: cardiac depression, arrhythmias, peaked P wave, depressed T wave HyperK+: cardiac excitability, fibrillation, DEATH, depressed P wave, peaked T waves,	3.2-5.2

- • Imaging
  - o EKG-if >40y.o., history of MI, HTN, CHF, SOB, HLD, angina
  - o CXR-if >60y.o. or >40y.o. w/ lung disease (COPD), CHF, smoker, pneumonia
    - ▪ Cervical XR-if RA
- • Pregnancy test if <50 yo
- • IV
  - o With NaCl—no sugar, for diabetics

- o   With lactated ringers—contains sugars, <u>for non diabetics</u>
  - o   80mL/hr
  - •   NPO status
- o   NO milk/solids 6-8 hours before surgery
- o   ALLOWED:
  - ☐   clear liquids 2-4 hrs preoperatively
  - ☐   "light" breakfast in the morning if surgery is in the afternoon
  - ☐   routine medications
  - ☐   breast milk/formula in pediatrics <2 y.o.

INTRAOPERATIVE:
Tourniquet settings

	Set pressure above systolic	Recommended max inflation time
UE	50mmHg	60 minutes
LE	100mmHg	90 minutes

Suturing

Horizontal mattress: sutures will be parallel to incision line
Vertical mattress: sutures will be horizontal to incision line
- •   The outer stitches pull on the deeper tissue
- •   The inner stitches pull on the superficial tissue

Complications:
- •   <u>Suture abscess</u>—cellulitis under the suture, red, swollen
- o   <u>Wound dehiscence</u>—2/2 to WB, trauma, infection
- •   <u>Dog ear</u>—treat by extending incision along dog ear to rotate flap, remove flap.

POSTOPERATIVE
Pearls:

BM, flatus, N/V/F/C, CP, calf pain, wiggle toes, sensation,

-Pain medication

- Suture removal: Dorsal foot: 2 weeks (10-14 days)

- Edema can remain for a year

- Hypotension normal due to blood loss

- Drains: <u>closed suction drain</u>-reduce hematoma and infection

5 W's (postop fever):

Timing	Post op fever	Disease	Treatment
<24 hours	Wind	atelectasis (from muscle relaxers), aspiration PNA	Incentive spirometry, CXR
@24 hours	Water	UTI	Straight catheter, UA, ABx
@48 hours	Walking	PE, DVT	TEDS stocking, SCD, walking, heparin
@72 hours	Wound	infection	culture, antibiotics, XR
Anytime	Wonder	wonder drugs	d/c drug or reverse drug

Infection

increased risk due to: smoking, DMARDs, TNF alpha inhibitors
Chlorhexadine is not superior to bar soap
Scrub brush is not necessary

Starchless gloves decrease infection rate
prevented by: hair removal, dental prophylaxis, pre-operative antibiotics infused within 1 hour of incision and finish before tourniquet inflated

Hematoma
ET:
- Collection of blood in closed tissue space due to:
  - Traumatic surgical dissection, poor hemostasis, creation of dead space, exposed cancellous bone, anticoagulation, improper bandaging
- Can lead to infection, long term swelling, pain, inflammation

TX:
Early
- Extravasation-remove a stitch and expel fluid
  - Aspiration-using needle
  - Steroid injection-decrease inflammation and pain
  - Wound re-entry-wound drained, bleeders ligated, drain inserted

Late
- Gentle heat-accelerate enzymatic degradation of hematoma
- Physical therapy-break up hematoma and encourage resorption

White toe
CP: white, cold to touch
ET: ARTERIAL ischemia
TX: STOP ice and elevation, loosen dressings, massage, heat pack to back, foot in dependent position, twist K wire, local anesthetic (topical or block)

Blue toe
CP: blue digit, warm to touch
ET: Due to VENOUS insufficiency
TX: same as white toe

Bioinformatics

Likelihood ratio
How many times more likely:
Probability of individual WITH condition having test result / probability of individual WITHOUT condition having test result

Confidence interval
A smaller confidence interval means a smaller range to be most accurate to a sample
- Smaller variation = smaller confidence interval
  - Larger sample = smaller confidence interval

Types of studies
1) Experimental study
   - You can *artificially* control (manipulate) every aspect
2) Observational study (clinical study)
   - Cannot control every detail
   - Level 1, 2, 3, 4, 5, case study, RCT

Types of bias
- Measurement bias-huge in experimental study, eliminated by calibrating the measurement devices
- Selection/sampling bias-error in choosing subjects for a study
- Funding bias
- Reporting bias
- Exclusion bias

Type 1 error-when one rejects null hypothesis when it is true. The probability of type 1 error is the level of significant of the test of hypothesis, known as alpha

Type 2 error-when one accepts null hypothesis when it is false.

Pain and functioning measurements:
- AOFAS score (American orthopaedic foot and ankle score)
- FAAM (foot and ankle activity measures)
- Foot-SANE (foot single assessment and numerical evaluation)

ANOVA-variance among different groups
1. For comparisons of 3+ (height between males, females, transgender)
   - Categorical vs continuous (numerical, infinite possibilities)
   - For parametric outcomes—those with a normal bell curve (height, not change in pocket)

T test-For comparisons of 2 (height between males and females)

Vocabulary terms

internal validity	degree to which results of a study is applicable to current study
external validity	degree to which results of study is applicable to other settings
prevalence	who had disease to begin with all cases at a time / population
incidence	NEW cases new cases / population
epidemic	localized
pandemic	global, more widespread
nominal data	no order (Blood type)
ordinal data	order matters but cannot quantify difference between each value (VAS)
interval data	continuous-i.e. temperature discrete-# residents
validity	same as accuracy how well data measures what it intended
reliability	reproducibility
responsiveness	results change as conditions change (GPA vs class rank in measuring academic success)
interpretability	can be easily compared relative to other results
how many between 1 SD vs 2 SD	1 SD 2/3, 2 SD 95%
regression to the mean	repeating tests would cause values to trend to the mean

181

long latency	time between exposure to risk and manifestation of disease
immediate vs distant cause	how likely does a risk cause the disease
common exposure to risk factor	i.e. cell phone radiation
low incidence of disease	not as bad as risk claims
calibration	how well does a risk represent **GROUP**
discrimination	how well does risk represent **INDIVIDUAL**
absolute risk	100/250 people die (GROUP)
attributable risk	
relative risk	23x more likely to die (INDIVIDUAL)
case report limit	<10 pts
sensitvitiy	people with the disease who test positive
specifcity	those without the disease who test negative
principal of equipoise	ethical when there's no clear evidence one is better than other
Hawthorne effect	patients perform differently when being experimented on
Efficacy	treatment under IDEAL circumstance
Effectiveness	treatment under REALITY
intention to treat trial	look at all 100 pts who began trial
explanatory trial	look at 50/100 pts after 50 dropped out
superiority trial	show one tx better than other
non-inferiority trial	new tx is is just as good
type 1 error	false **positive**
type 2 error	false **negative**
p value	STATISTICAL SIGNFICANCE difference in tx not due to chance. need value at least 0.05. lower p value is better does not equal clinical significant (need to evaluate cost, etc)
Parametric test	follows BELL CURVE
null hypothesis	researcher tries to disprove

alternative hypothesis	researcher tries to PROVE
prevalance screen	FIRST TIME screening performed
incidence screen	TIME PERIOD screening performed
length time bias	Identify diseases with inherent good prognosis i.e. screening for breast CA
Standard error of mean	Estimate of standard deviation by taking a smaller sample size

References

1. Brand, Paul W. "Tenderizing the foot." Foot & ankle international 24.6 (2003): 457-461.
2. Lavery, Lawrence A., et al. "Risk factors for foot infections in individuals with diabetes." Diabetes care 29.6 (2006): 1288-1293.
3. Singh, Nalini, David G. Armstrong, and Benjamin A. Lipsky. "Preventing foot ulcers in patients with diabetes." Jama 293.2 (2005): 217-228.
4. Lavery, Lawrence A., et al. "Validation of the Infectious Diseases Society of America's diabetic foot infection classification system." Clinical infectious diseases 44.4 (2007): 562-565
5. Waters, R. L., et al. "Energy cost of walking of amputees: the influence of level of amputation." The Journal of Bone & Joint Surgery 58.1 (1976): 42-46.
6. Jupiter, Daniel C., et al. "The impact of foot ulceration and amputation on mortality in diabetic patients. I: From ulceration to death, a systematic review." International wound journal (2015).
7. Apelqvist J, Larsson J, Agardh CD. Long-term prognosis for diabetic patients with foot ulcers. J Intern Med 1993;233:485 – 91.
8. Lee JS, Lu M, Lee VS, Russel D, Bahr C, Lee ET. Lower extremity amputation: incidence, risk factors, and mortality in the Oklahoma Indian diabetes study. Diabetes 42:876–882, 1993.
9. Lavery et al, Effectiveness of the Diabetic Foot Risk Classification System of the International Working Group on the Diabetic foot, Diabetes Care 2001, 24; 8:1442-47
10. Lavery, Lawrence A., David G. Armstrong, and Lawrence B. Harkless. "Classification of diabetic foot wounds." The Journal of foot and ankle surgery 35.6 (1996): 528-531.
11. Brownlee, Michael. "The pathobiology of diabetic complications a unifying mechanism." Diabetes 54.6 (2005): 1615-1625.
12. Cavanagh PR et al, Nonsurgical Strategies for Healing and Preventing Recurrence of Diabetic Foot Ulcers, Foot Ankle Clinics, 2006, 735-743
13. Brand, Paul W. "Tenderizing the foot." Foot & ankle international 24.6 (2003): 457-461

14. Armstrong, David G., et al. "Skin temperature monitoring reduces the risk for diabetic foot ulceration in high-risk patients." The American journal of medicine 120.12 (2007): 1042-1046

15. Armstrong, David G., et al. "Quality of life in healing diabetic wounds: does the end justify the means?." The Journal of Foot and Ankle Surgery 47.4 (2008): 278-282.

16. Caputo, Gregory M., et al. "Assessment and management of foot disease in patients with diabetes." New England Journal of Medicine 331.13 (1994): 854-860

17. Gutekunst, David J., et al. "Removable cast walker boots yield greater forefoot off-loading than total contact casts." Clinical Biomechanics 26.6 (2011): 649-654.

18. Sheehan, Peter, et al. "Percent change in wound area of diabetic foot ulcers over a 4-week period is a robust predictor of complete healing in a 12-week prospective trial." Diabetes care 26.6 (2003): 1879-1882.

19. Zimny, Stefan, Helmut Schatz, and Martin Pfohl. "Determinants and estimation of healing times in diabetic foot ulcers." Journal of Diabetes and its Complications 16.5 (2002): 327-332

20. Löndahl, Magnus, et al. "Hyperbaric oxygen therapy facilitates healing of chronic foot ulcers in patients with diabetes." Diabetes care 33.5 (2010): 998-1003

21. van Schie, Carine, et al. "Design criteria for rigid rocker shoes." Foot & Ankle International 21.10 (2000): 833-844

22. Lipsky, Benjamin A., et al. "2012 Infectious Diseases Society of America clinical practice guideline for the diagnosis and treatment of diabetic foot infections." Clinical infectious diseases 54.12 (2012): e132-e173

23. Zenelaj, Besa, et al. "Do Diabetic Foot Infections With Methicillin-Resistant Staphylococcus aureus Differ From Those With Other Pathogens?." The international journal of lower extremity wounds (2014): 1534734614550311.

24. Brucato, Maryellen P., Krupa Patel, and Obinna Mgbako. "Diagnosis of Gas Gangrene: Does a Discrepancy Exist between the Published Data and Practice." The Journal of Foot and Ankle Surgery 53.2 (2014): 137-140.

25. Lipsky, Benjamin A., et al. "2012 Infectious Diseases Society of America clinical practice guideline for the diagnosis and treatment of diabetic foot infections." Clinical infectious diseases 54.12 (2012): e132-e173.

26. Zaulyanov, Larissa, and Robert S. Kirsner. "A review of a bi-layered living cell treatment (Apligraf®) in the treatment of venous leg ulcers and diabetic foot ulcers." Clinical interventions in aging 2.1 (2007): 93

27. Brown B, Lindberg K, Reing J, Stolz DB, Badylak SF. The basement membrane component of biologic scaffolds derived from extracellular matrix. Tissue Eng 2006;12:519–26.

28. Lavery, Lawrence A., et al. "The efficacy and safety of Grafix® for the treatment of chronic diabetic foot ulcers: results of a multi-centre, controlled, randomised, blinded, clinical trial." International wound journal 11.5 (2014): 554-560.

29. Garwood, Caitlin S., John S. Steinberg, and Paul J. Kim. "Bioengineered Alternative Tissues in Diabetic Wound Healing." Clinics in podiatric medicine and surgery 32.1 (2015): 121-133.

30. A clinical staging system for adult osteomyelitis. CORR. 2003; (414): 7-24

31. Grayson, M. Lindsay, et al. "Probing to bone in infected pedal ulcers: a clinical sign of underlying osteomyelitis in diabetic patients." Jama 273.9 (1995): 721-723.

32. Lavery, Lawrence A., et al. "Probe-to-Bone Test for Diagnosing Diabetic Foot Osteomyelitis Reliable or relic?." Diabetes care 30.2 (2007): 270-274.

33. Shone, Alison, et al. "Probing the validity of the probe-to-bone test in the diagnosis of osteomyelitis of the foot in diabetes." Diabetes Care 29.4 (2006): 945-945.

34. Thorning, Chandani, et al. "Midfoot and hindfoot bone marrow edema identified by magnetic resonance imaging in feet of subjects with diabetes and neuropathic ulceration is common but of unknown clinical significance." Diabetes care 33.7 (2010): 1602-1603.

35. Tone, Alina, et al. "Six-Week Versus Twelve-Week Antibiotic Therapy for Nonsurgically Treated Diabetic Foot Osteomyelitis: A Multicenter Open-Label Controlled Randomized Study." Diabetes care 38.2 (2015): 302-307.

36. Seddon, H. J. "A classification of nerve injuries." British medical journal 2.4260 (1942): 237.

37. Sunderland, Sydney, and Francis Walshe. "Nerves and nerve injuries." (1968): 9.

38. Martyn CN, Hughes RAC. Epidemiology of peripheral neuropathy. J Neurol Neu- rosurg Psychiatry. 1997 Apr;62(4):310-8.

39. Faldini, Cesare, et al. "Surgical Treatment of Cavus Foot in Charcot-Marie-Tooth Disease: A Review of Twenty-four Cases." The Journal of Bone & Joint Surgery 97.6 (2015): e30.

40. Eichenholtz SN. Charcot Joints, p7-8, Springfield, Illinois, Charles C Thomas, 1966

41. de Souza, Leo J. "Charcot arthropathy and immobilization in a weight-bearing total contact cast." The Journal of Bone & Joint Surgery 90.4 (2008): 754-759.

42. Rogers, Lee C., et al. "The Charcot foot in diabetes." Diabetes Care 34.9 (2011): 2123-2129

43. Brodsky JW. The diabetic foot. In: Coughlin and Mann's 1992 edition

44. Charcot neuroarthropathy of the foot and ankle. CORR. 1998; 349: 116-131

45. Thomson, Colin E., J. N. Gibson, and Denis Martin. "Interventions for the treatment of Morton's neuroma." The Cochrane Library (2004).

46. Arroyo Cl, Tritto VG, Buchbinder D, et al. Optimal waiting period for foot salvage surgery following limb revascularization. J Foot Ankle Surg. 2002;41(4):228-32.

47. Mills, Joseph L., et al. "The Society for Vascular Surgery lower extremity threatened limb classification system: risk stratification based on Wound, Ischemia, and foot Infection (WIfI)." Journal of vascular surgery 59.1 (2014): 220-234.

48. Fleischer, Adam E., et al. "American College of Foot and Ankle Surgeons' Clinical Consensus Statement: Risk, Prevention, and Diagnosis of Venous Thromboembolism Disease in Foot and Ankle Surgery and Injuries Requiring Immobilization." The Journal of Foot and Ankle Surgery (2015).

49. Crawford F, Hollis S "Topical treatments for fungal infections of the skin and nails of the foot." The Cochrane Library 2007

50.   Bell-Syer, Sally EM, et al. "Oral treatments for fungal infections of the skin of the foot." The Cochrane Library (2012)

51.   Gupta R, Gupta S. Topical adapalene in the treatment of plantar warts; randomized comparative open trial in comparison with cryotherapy. Indian J Dermatol. 2015; 60(1):102.

52.   Images taken from Christman, Robert. Foot and ankle radiology. Lippincott Williams & Wilkins, 2014.

53.   Johnson, Cherie H., and Jeffrey C. Christensen. "Biomechanics of the first ray part V: The effect of equinus deformity: A 3-dimensional kinematic study on a cadaver model." The Journal of foot and ankle surgery 44.2 (2005): 114-120.

54.   Sanicola, Shawn M., Thomas B. Arnold, and Lawrence Osher. "Is the radiographic appearance of the hallucal tarsometatarsal joint representative of its true anatomical structure?." Journal of the American Podiatric Medical Association 92.9 (2002): 491-498.

55.   Miller, SJ THE FIRST METATARSOCUNEIFORM JOINT: Analysis and Clinical Application, Podiatry Institute Update 1995

56.   Okuda, Ryuzo, et al. "The shape of the lateral edge of the first metatarsal head as a risk factor for recurrence of hallux valgus." The Journal of Bone & Joint Surgery 89.10 (2007): 2163-2172.

57.   Okuda, Ryuzo, et al. "The shape of the lateral edge of the first metatarsal head as a risk factor for recurrence of hallux valgus." The Journal of Bone & Joint Surgery 89.10 (2007): 2163-2172.

58.   Lundgren, P., et al. "Invasive in vivo measurement of rear-, mid-and forefoot motion during walking." Gait & posture 28.1 (2008): 93-100.

59.   Roling, Brian A., Jeffrey C. Christensen, and Cherie H. Johnson. "Biomechanics of the first ray. Part IV: the effect of selected medial column arthrodeses. A three-dimensional kinematic analysis in a cadaver model." The Journal of foot and ankle surgery 41.5 (2002): 278-285

60.   Torkki, Markus, et al. "Surgery vs orthosis vs watchful waiting for hallux valgus: a randomized controlled trial." Jama 285.19 (2001): 2474-2480.

61.   Okuda, Ryuzo, et al. "Postoperative incomplete reduction of the sesamoids as a risk factor for recurrence of hallux valgus." The Journal of Bone & Joint Surgery 91.7 (2009): 1637-1645.

62.   Dayton, Paul, Merrell Kauwe, and Mindi Feilmeier. "Is Our Current Paradigm for Evaluation and Management of the Bunion Deformity Flawed? A Discussion of Procedure Philosophy Relative to Anatomy." The Journal of Foot and Ankle Surgery 54.1 (2015): 102-111.

63.   Vanore et al, Diagnosis and Treatment of First Metatarsophalangeal Joint Disorders. Section 1: Hallux Valgus, Journal of Foot and Ankle Surgery 2003, 42; 3:112-23

64.   Ryan, Jay D., Eugene D. Timpano, and Thomas A. Brosky. "Average Depth of Tarsometatarsal Joint for Trephine Arthrodesis." The Journal of Foot and Ankle Surgery 51.2 (2012): 168-171.

65.   Coughlin, Michael J., and Paul S. Shurnas. "Hallux rigidus." The Journal of Bone & Joint Surgery 85.11 (2003): 2072-2088

66.   Bouaicha, Samy, et al. "Radiographic analysis of metatarsus primus elevatus and hallux rigidus." Foot & ankle international 31.9 (2010): 807-814

67.   Christman, Robert A., et al. "Radiographic analysis of metatarsus primus elevatus: a preliminary study." Journal of the American Podiatric Medical Association 91.6 (2001): 294-299. APA

68.   Roukis, Thomas S. "Metatarsus primus elevatus in hallux rigidus: fact or fiction?." Journal of the American Podiatric Medical Association 95.3 (2005): 221-228

69.   Coughlin, Michael J., and Paul S. Shurnas. "Hallux rigidus." The Journal of Bone & Joint Surgery 85.11 (2003): 2072-2088

70.   Cronin, John J., et al. "Intermetatarsal angle after first metatarsophalangeal joint arthrodesis for hallux valgus." Foot & ankle international 27.2 (2006): 104-109

71.   Kline, Alex J., and Carl T. Hasselman. "Metatarsal head resurfacing for advanced hallux rigidus." Foot & ankle international (2013): 1071100713478930.

72.   Vanore et al, Diagnosis and Treatment of First Metatarsophalangeal Joint Disorders. Section 2: Hallux Rigidus, Journal of Foot and Ankle Surgery 2003, 42; 3:124-36

73.   Vanore et al, Diagnosis and Treatment of First Metatarsophalangeal Joint Disorders. Section 2: Hallux Rigidus, Journal of Foot and Ankle Surgery 2003, 42; 3:124-36

74.   Canales, Michael B., et al. "Fact or Fiction? Iatrogenic Hallux Abducto Valgus Secondary to Tibial Sesamoidectomy." The Journal of Foot and Ankle Surgery 54.1 (2015): 82-88

75.   Hunter, Joshua G., et al. "Risk Factors for Failure of a Single Surgical Debridement in Adults with Acute Septic Arthritis." The Journal of Bone & Joint Surgery 97.7 (2015): 558-564.

76.   JOHNSON, KENNETH A., and DAVID E. STROM. "Tibialis posterior tendon dysfunction." Clinical orthopaedics and related research 239 (1989): 196-206.

77.   Bluman, Eric M., Craig I. Title, and Mark S. Myerson. "Posterior tibial tendon rupture: a refined classification system." Foot and ankle clinics 12.2 (2007): 233-249

78.   Shibuya, Naohiro, Ryan T. Kitterman, and Daniel C. Jupiter. "Evaluation of the Rearfoot Component (Module 3) of the ACFAS Scoring Scale." The Journal of Foot and Ankle Surgery 53.5 (2014): 544-547.

79.   Labovitz, Jonathan M. "The algorithmic approach to pediatric flexible pes planovalgus." Clinics in podiatric medicine and surgery 23.1 (2006): 57-76

80.   Funk, DANIEL A., J. R. Cass, and K. A. Johnson. "Acquired adult flat foot secondary to posterior tibial-tendon pathology." The Journal of Bone & Joint Surgery 68.1 (1986): 95-102.

81.   Conti, Stephen, James Michelson, and Melvin Jahss. "Clinical significance of magnetic resonance imaging in preoperative planning for reconstruction of posterior tibial tendon ruptures." Foot & Ankle International 13.4 (1992): 208-214

82.   Lawson, J. P., et al. "The painful accessory navicular." Skeletal radiology 12.4 (1984): 250-262

83.   Astion, Donna J., et al. "Motion of the Hindfoot after Simulated Arthrodesis*." The Journal of Bone & Joint Surgery 79.2 (1997): 241-6

84.   Brewerton DA, Sandifer PH, Sweetnam DR. "Idiopathic" pes cavus: an investi- gation into its aetiology. Br Med J. 1963 Sep 14;2(5358):659-61.

85. Burns, Joshua, et al. "Interventions for the prevention and treatment of pes cavus." The Cochrane Library (2007)
86. Lundgren, P., et al. "Invasive in vivo measurement of rear-, mid-and forefoot motion during walking." Gait & posture 28.1 (2008): 93-100.
87. Janssen KW, Hendriks MR, van Mechelen W, Verhagen E. The cost-effectiveness of measures to prevent recurrent ankle sprains: results of a 3-arm randomized con- trolled trial. Am J Sports Med. 2014 Apr 21;42(7):1534-41. Kwon, John Y., et al. "A Cadaver Study Revisiting the Original Methodology of Lauge-Hansen and a Commentary on Modern Usage." The Journal of Bone & Joint Surgery 97.7 (2015): 604-609

88. Bucholz, Robert W., et al. Rockwood and Green's Fractures in Adults: Rockwood, Green, and Wilkins' Fractures. Lippincott Williams & Wilkins, 2002.
89. Yablon, ISADORE G., F. G. Heller, and L. E. R. O. Y. Shouse. "The key role of the lateral malleolus in displaced fractures of the ankle." The Journal of Bone & Joint Surgery 59.2 (1977): 169-173.
90. Ramsey, PAUL L., and W. I. L. L. I. A. M. HAMIlTON. "Changes in tibiotalar area of contact caused by lateral talar shift." The Journal of Bone & Joint Surgery 58.3 (1976): 356-357.
91. Zindrick, M. R., et al. "The effect of lateral talar shift upon the biomechanics of the ankle joint." Orthop Trans 9 (1985): 332-333.
92. Stuart, Kyle, and Vinod K. Panchbhavi. "The fate of syndesmotic screws." Foot & ankle international 32.5 (2011): 519-525.
93. Ostrum, Robert F., and Alan S. Litsky. "Tension band fixation of medial malleolus fractures." Journal of orthopaedic trauma 6.4 (1992): 464-468.
94. Haraguchi, Naoki, et al. "Pathoanatomy of posterior malleolar fractures of the ankle." The Journal of Bone & Joint Surgery 88.5 (2006): 1085-1092.
95. Gardner MJ, et al., Clin Orthop Rel Res. 447:165-71, 2006.
96. Starkweather, Michael P., David R. Collman, and John M. Schuberth. "Early protected weightbearing after open reduction internal fixation of ankle fractures." The Journal of Foot and Ankle Surgery 51.5 (2012): 575-578
97. Ogilvie-Harris, D. J., S. C. Reed, and T. P. Hedman. "Disruption of the ankle syndesmosis: biomechanical study of the ligamentous restraints." Arthroscopy: The Journal of Arthroscopic & Related Surgery 10.5 (1994): 558-560.
98. Yamaguchi, Ken, et al. "Operative treatment of syndesmotic disruptions without use of a syndesmotic screw: a prospective clinical study." Foot & Ankle International 15.8 (1994): 407-414.
99. Tornetta III, Paul, et al. "Overtightening of the ankle syndesmosis: is it really possible?." The Journal of Bone & Joint Surgery 83.4 (2001): 489-489.
100. Kennedy, J. G., et al. "Evaluation of the syndesmotic screw in low Weber C ankle fractures." Journal of orthopaedic trauma 14.5 (2000): 359-366.
101. Yamaguchi, Ken, et al. "Operative treatment of syndesmotic disruptions without use of a syndesmotic screw: a prospective clinical study." Foot & Ankle International 15.8 (1994): 407-414.
102. Beumer, Annechien, et al. "Screw fixation of the syndesmosis: a cadaver model comparing stainless steel and titanium screws and three and four cortical fixation." Injury 36.1 (2005): 60-64.
103. Thompson, Michael C., and Dirk S. Gesink. "Biomechanical comparison of syndesmosis fixation with 3.5-and 4.5-millimeter stainless steel screws." Foot & Ankle International 21.9 (2000): 736-741.
104. Beumer, Annechien, et al. "Screw fixation of the syndesmosis: a cadaver model comparing stainless steel and titanium screws and three and four cortical fixation." Injury 36.1 (2005): 60-64.
105. Naqvi GA1, Am J Sports Med. 2012 Dec;40(12):2828-35.
106. Coughlin, Michael J., Charles L. Saltzman, and Roger A. Mann. Mann's Surgery of the Foot and Ankle: Expert Consult-Online. Elsevier Health Sciences, 2013.
107. Ling, Jeffrey S., et al. "Investigating the Relationship Between Ankle Arthrodesis and Adjacent-Joint Arthritis in the Hindfoot." The Journal of Bone & Joint Surgery 97.6 (2015): 513-519.
108. Nguyen, Mai P., et al. "Intermediate-Term Follow-up After Ankle Distraction for Treatment of End-Stage Osteoarthritis." The Journal of Bone & Joint Surgery 97.7 (2015): 590-596.
109. Gupta, Sanjeev, J. Kent Ellington, and Mark S. Myerson. "Management of specific complications after revision total ankle replacement." Seminars in Arthroplasty. Vol. 21. No. 4. WB Saunders, 2010.
110. Patel, Amar, and Benedict DiGiovanni. "Association between plantar fasciitis and isolated contracture of the gastrocnemius." Foot & ankle international 32.1 (2011): 5-8.
111. Harty, James, et al. "The role of hamstring tightness in plantar fasciitis." Foot & ankle international 26.12 (2005): 1089-1092.
112. Digiovanni, Benedict F., et al. "Plantar fascia-specific stretching exercise improves outcomes in patients with chronic plantar fasciitis." The Journal of Bone and Joint Surgery 88.8 (2006): 1775-1781.
113. Maffulli N, Papalia R, D'Adamio S, Diaz Balzani L, Denaro V. Pharmacological interventions for the treatment of Achilles tendinopathy: a systematic review of randomized controlled trials. Br Med Bull. 2015 Mar;113(1):101-15. Epub 2015 Jan 12.
114. Saltzman CL, Tearse DS. Achilles tendon injuries. J Am Acad Orthop Surg. 1998 Sep-Oct;6(5):316-25.
115. Willits, Kevin, et al. "Operative versus nonoperative treatment of acute Achilles tendon ruptures." The Journal of Bone & Joint Surgery 92.17 (2010): 2767-2775.
116. Soroceanu A, et al. J Bone Joint Surg Am. 2012 Dec 5;94(23):2136-43.
117. Wilkins R, Bisson LJ. Am J Sports Med. 2012 Sep;40(9):2154-60.
118. Uquillas, Carlos A., et al. "Everything Achilles: Knowledge Update and Current Concepts in Management." J Bone Joint Surg Am 97.14 (2015): 1187-1195.
119. DeVries, J. George, et al. "The Fifth Metatarsal Base: Anatomic Evaluation Regarding Fracture Mechanism and Treatment Algorithms." The Journal of Foot and Ankle Surgery 54.1 (2015): 94-98
120. Scott, Ryan T., Christopher F. Hyer, and Shyler L. DeMill. "Screw Fixation Diameter for Fifth Metatarsal Jones Fracture: A Cadaveric Study." The Journal of Foot and Ankle Surgery (2015)

121. http://www.podiatrytoday.com/rethinking-our-approach-jones-fractures-facilitate-shorter-post-op-recovery
122. DeVries, J. George, et al. "The Fifth Metatarsal Base: Anatomic Evaluation Regarding Fracture Mechanism and Treatment Algorithms." The Journal of Foot and Ankle Surgery 54.1 (2015): 94-98
123. Lee SK, Park JS, Choy WS. Locking compression plate distal ulna hook plate as alternative fixation for fifth metatarsal base fracture. J Foot Ankle Surg 53:522–528, 2014.
124. Bruce J, Sutherland A. Cochrane Database Syst Rev. 2013 Jan 31;1:CD008628.
125. Buckley, Richard, et al. "Operative compared with nonoperative treatment of displaced intra-articular calcaneal fractures." The Journal of Bone & Joint Surgery 84.10 (2002): 1733-1744.
126. Radiology and Biomechanical Foot Types, Donald R. Green, Podiatry Institute Update, 1998
127. Seibel, Michael O. Foot Function: A programmed text. Williams & Wilkins, 1988
128. Stauffer, Richard N., Edward YS Chao, and Robert C. Brewster. "Force and motion analysis of the normal, diseased, and prosthetic ankle joint." Clinical orthopaedics and related research 127 (1977): 189-196.
129. Nigg, Benno M et al "Shoe inserts and orthotics for sport and physical activities." Medicine and science in sports and exercise 31 (1999): S421-S428
130. http://www.prolaborthotics.com/Education/TermsandDefinitions/tabid/85/Default.aspx
131. Stevens, Dennis L., et al. "Practice guidelines for the diagnosis and management of skin and soft tissue infections: 2014 update by the Infectious Diseases Society of America." Clinical Infectious Diseases 59.2 (2014): e10-e52.
132. Astion, Donna J., et al. "Motion of the Hindfoot after Simulated Arthrodesis*." The Journal of Bone & Joint Surgery 79.2 (1997): 241-6.
133. Trevino, Saul, Mark Gibbs, and Vinod Panchbhavi. "Evaluation of results of endoscopic gastrocnemius recession." Foot & ankle international 26.5 (2005): 359-364.
134. Roukis, Thomas S., and Monica H. Schweinberger. "Complications associated with uni-portal endoscopic gastrocnemius recession in a diabetic patient population: an observational case series." The journal of Foot and Ankle Surgery 49.1 (2010): 68-70.

Made in the USA
San Bernardino, CA
26 November 2016